Benno ter Kuile
Editor

Antimicrobial Resistance and Antibiotics Usage in Livestock

Why Prevention Must Start on the Farm

Springer

Editor
Benno ter Kuile
Universiteit van Amsterdam
Amsterdam, The Netherlands

ISBN 978-3-032-04597-3 ISBN 978-3-032-04598-0 (eBook)
https://doi.org/10.1007/978-3-032-04598-0

This Springer imprint is published by the registered company Springer Nature Switzerland AG
The registered company address is: Gewerbestrasse 11, 6330 Cham, Switzerland

Foreword

Food safety has many aspects. One of these is antimicrobial resistance. The resistance that is selected in the livestock sector and is transferred to human pathogens is by law considered a zoonosis. In the Netherlands, the Office for Risk Assessment & Research (BuRO) is responsible for advising policymakers and law enforcement on how to reduce the risks for human health care caused by usage of antimicrobials in livestock. To give solid advice, a thorough understanding of the issues is indispensable. In order to obtain a state-of-the-art overview of the scientific knowledge concerning antibiotic resistance in the veterinary sector, BuRO organized a conference bringing together experts from all over the world to discuss measures that will allow to treat infectious diseases in livestock with minimal negative consequences for public health. This conference took place in Amsterdam on October 5 and 6, 2023. The outcome was used by participating experts to write reviews on the subjects that comprise the core of this issue.

The result is a book that is far more than a conference book. It also contains chapters of a more general character that provide an overview of antimicrobial resistance from the perspective of food safety. While the opinions viewed at the conference have inspired the authors and helped to ascertain completeness, they are also thoroughly researched and referenced. The first chapter provides a general background and is followed by a chapter discussing preventive measures to minimize the impact of antimicrobial usage for livestock on overall antibiotic resistance. The effects of antimicrobials discarded in the environment on development and spreading of resistance are evaluated in the third chapter. The fourth chapter deals with the spread of antimicrobial resistance caused by food and animal movements. Fluoroquinolones are the subject of Chap. 5. The last two chapters take the EU laws and regulations as example of rules for the veterinary application of antimicrobials and the actual implementation thereof.

The combination of the basic science and the application for policymaking and law enforcement make this book very useful for everybody who busies him-/herself with antimicrobial resistance, either as a scientist, health expert, or policymaker. The simple problems related to antibiotic resistance have long been solved and the low-hanging fruits have been harvested. Still, better methods of application and more effectively focused efforts can reduce the risks caused by antimicrobial resistance at acceptable costs for society. Pointing out these better methods and providing the scientific basis is the purpose of this book. As a risk-assessor I will certainly use it and I expect that many of my colleagues will do so too.

Dick Sijm
Director, Office for Risk Assessment & Research
The Netherlands Food and Consumer Product Safety Authority,
Utrecht, The Netherlands

Competing Interests

The authors declare that no competing interests exist.

Ethics Approval Not applicable

About the Book

This book was conceived during the scientific conference on

"Optimal practices to protect human health care from antimicrobial resistance selected in the veterinary domain"

Antimicrobial resistance (AMR) is recognized as a major public health threat. From a legal point of view the resistance that is selected by usage of antibiotics for livestock and subsequently transferred to human pathogens is considered a zoonosis. In many countries, legislation demanding measures to prevent development and spreading of antibiotic resistance in the veterinary sector has been implemented successfully. By now, most of the low-hanging fruits have already been harvested with respect to controlling and reducing antimicrobial resistance in the livestock sector. Furthermore, the measures to be applied are at least known, if not yet implemented. On October 5 and 6, 2023, a conference was held in Amsterdam, The Netherlands, to deliberate potential next steps. The aim of the conference was to discuss innovative additional measures to prevent development of resistance in pathogens and commensal bacteria of animals. In addition, the 83 participants, all with backgrounds in antimicrobial resistance, explored possibilities to prevent transfer to human health care after selection has taken place.

The conference program consisted of both lectures and interactive breakout sessions and was intended for researchers as well as for policymakers involved in the battle against antimicrobial resistance. The results of the breakout sessions are presented in the chapters of this book. The chairs of each session converted the consensus into a short review on the subject and these were combined into chapters. These extended session reports are accompanied by a review introduction and chapters on the EU Regulations 2019/4 and 2019/6 as examples of legislation that provides law enforcement agencies with effective tools to combat antimicrobial resistance. The following subjects were discussed in these breakout sessions:

- Hygiene, animal health and animal welfare
- Impact of antimicrobial usage on AMR prevalence
- Alternative treatments to reduce the need for antimicrobials

- How to measure the outcome of preventive measures
- Consequences of antimicrobial residues in the environment
- Food as transmission route for resistance
- Spreading resistance through animal transfer
- Improving farm management in the context of AMR
- Wildlife as possible transmission route
- Application of critically important antimicrobials

These sessions form the basis for Chaps. 2, 3, and 4. Chapter 1 provides an overview, Chap. 5 reviews specific aspects of fluoroquinolones, and Chaps. 6 and 7 expand on the EU legislation and its implementation. Taken together the various types of information provide a perspective for actions and measures to counter resistance.

Contents

About the Editor

Benno ter Kuile has been a policymaker and researcher on the subject of antimicrobial resistance since 2001. Before that he had an academic career in microbiology and protozoology. Working for the Office for Risk Assessment & Research of The Netherlands Food and Consumer Product Safety Authority and the legal predecessors, he needed more information than was available on the relationship between exposure to antimicrobials and the development and spreading of antibiotic resistance. Therefore, he started a research group at the University of Amsterdam focusing on that subject. He later became a full professor there on the subject of antimicrobial resistance in the food chain. He has (co-)authored some 50 articles on the subject and is associate editor for two journals, specializing on the topic of antibiotic resistance.

Chapter 1
Overview and Background: Antimicrobial Resistance in the Veterinary Sector

Benno ter Kuile

Abstract The costs of antimicrobial resistance developed in the livestock sector and spreading form there to human health care is considerable. Nowadays this problem is usually approached for the so-called One-Health perspective. Development of resistance is mostly the consequence of exposure to non-lethal concentrations of antibiotics, both when resistance genes on plasmids are involved and when resistance is induced *de novo*. Detailed analysis of the data on veterinary usage of antibiotics and prevalence of resistance suggest that the reduction of usage has caused a decrease of the percentage of resistance bacteria. Specific forms of resistance, such as multi-resistance and carbapenem resistance, still form a major threat for public health. Once resistance has been selected for in the veterinary sector, it is not effective to try to prevent it from reaching human health care. Reducing development of resistance at the source is more efficient.

Keywords Antimicrobial resistance · One-Health · Veterinary health care · AMR prevention

Introduction

The steady increase of resistance of microbes against antimicrobials is a generally recognized problem for public health (Chatterjee et al. 2018). Resistance is the effect of exposure to non-lethal concentrations of antibiotics, both for human health care and for treatment of infections in animals (Ter Kuile et al. 2016). In both sectors, resistance increase the costs of treating infections, as the means of first choice are no longer effective. Bacteria can become resistant to several and at times almost

B. ter Kuile (✉)
Department of Molecular Biology and Microbial Food Safety, Swammerdam Institute of Life Sciences, University of Amsterdam, Amsterdam, The Netherlands

The Netherlands Food and Consumer Products Safety Authority, Utrecht, The Netherlands
e-mail: b.h.terkuile@uva.nl

B. ter Kuile (ed.), *Antimicrobial Resistance and Antibiotics Usage in Livestock*,
https://doi.org/10.1007/978-3-032-04598-0_1

all antibiotics. Therefore, means of last resort are needed in such cases, which have more severe side-effects and are often more expensive (Huebner et al. 2019). When resistance originally selected in the veterinary sector migrates to the human health care, the costs for public health increase. In extreme cases, resistance can even develop against the antimicrobials serving as means of last resort, resulting in untreatable infections (Ho et al. 2025). The estimate is that for the entire EU, some 33,000 additional deaths occur and an extra cost for human health care of 1.5–3.5 billion euro (EU 2017; Cassini et al. 2019a; Freitas et al. 2020). There is not enough information available to make a more precise and better supported estimate and the methods of making such estimate are subject of dispute as well (Dunachie et al. 2020). The costs of raising animals for meat production increase as well, because treating infections in production animals becomes more expensive as well. There is no estimate for these costs, other than that the costs of not using any antibiotics at all when a cow stops giving milk to have another calf are around $ 60,- per cow per year (Lhermie et al. 2018a, b). Extrapolation of that amount would give an unrealistically high estimate for the veterinary sector of the costs of resistance.

Definitions and Terminology

The word "antibiotic" literally means "against life". The words "antibiotic' and "antimicrobial" are used interchangeably. A general definition is: "A drug used to treat infections caused by bacteria and other microorganisms". An alternative definition is: "a medicine that inhibits the growth of or destroys microorganisms". These can be natural compounds and derivatives thereof and completely synthetic molecules. There are some 210 natural antibiotics and around 500 derivatives (Berdy 2012). Antimicrobials are divided in classes according to structure and mechanism of operation. There is no consensus on this taxonomy, but usually 10 classes are distinguished. An important functional difference is between bactericidal and bacteriostatic antibiotics. The first kill the microbes, while the latter slow down growth. The difference is not clear-cut. At high concentration of bacteriostatic drugs, the cells die as well. The real difference seems to be that bacteriostatic compound slow down metabolism, while bactericidal drugs increase metabolic rates. (Qi et al. 2023a, b). Antimicrobials against eukaryotic micro-organisms are sometimes indicated as "anti-parasitics".

Antimicrobial resistance is a multi-faceted phenomenon. When a microbe is resistant against one antibiotic, it is usually also resistant against related compounds with the same working mechanism, but not always to the same degree (Ho et al. 2025). For example, a strain that is highly resistant against penicillin can be moderately resistant against the closely related drug amoxicillin. When the mechanisms of resistance are more complex, so does the overall response of the cell. Beta-lactam antibiotics can be disabled by enzymes of the extended spectrum beta-lactamase group or by the AmpC protein (Lima et al. 2020). Both classes of enzymes open the beta-lactam ring and thereby render the antibiotic ineffective. Several different genes can code for extended spectrum beta-lactamase (ESBL) proteins, that each result in a very similar genotype, but the ampC gene codes for a protein with more limited range that also is not always expressed. As a results, all antibiotics that are destroyed by AmpC are also disabled by ESBL's, but the opposite is not true. Hence, for monitoring purposes first the resistance profile is determined and when needed the diagnosis is confirmed by genotyping.

Genotyping is used to rapidly diagnose the risks connected to a specific bacterial strain. Whole genome sequencing (WGS) is applied with increasing frequency to map the presence of antimicrobial resistance genes and thereby predict the risks (Mustafa 2024). WGS identifies the presence of resistance genes, but does not predict whether these are expressed. The level of expression determines to which extent a microbe is resistant. The presence of a gene only indicates that there is a chance that an isolate can develop a certain type of resistance when exposed to the corresponding antibiotic. The minimal inhibiting concentration (MIC) of the strain for that antibiotic indicates the effectiveness of the resistance mechanisms against the antimicrobial. The higher the MIC, the more resistant the isolate.

Microorganisms can be resistant to 1 or several antibiotics, that do not by necessity belong to the same class. Resistance against 3 or more antibiotics is indicated with the term "multi-resistant". The number of resistances often depends on the history of exposure. In particular soil bacteria that are exposed to low concentrations of various antibiotics are at times resistant to more than 15 antibiotics (Walsh and Duffy 2013). Once a bacterium has become resistant against one drug, it can acquire the second resistance faster (Hoeksema et al. 2019). The reason for that is that in the first round the cells that become resistant are not only selected for the resistance itself, but also for the ability to become resistant. As a consequence, strains that are resistant against 1 or a few antibiotics, develop the next resistances much quicker. A related phenomenon is co-selection (Maurya et al. 2020). When a microbe is resistant against two or more antimicrobials and is exposed to one of these, then the other resistances will be selected as well and spread further.

Resistance of bacteria against antibiotics is not on/off, but gradual (EFSA-ECDC 2024). Even when a naïve wildtype is described as fully susceptible, it can still survive low concentrations of antimicrobials and grow when exposed to these. The MIC is the measure for sensitivity and is defined as the lowest concentration preventing growth of the microbe. This can be measured by two different methods. One is the diffusion disk (Jorgensen and Ferraro 2009), a thin disk from which antibiotics diffuse onto an agar plate is placed on a plate on which a thin culture has been spread. The extent of resistance is determined by measuring the zone in which growth is prevented (https://www.eucast.org/). This method is very suitable for large numbers of samples, but is not very precise. Worldwide it is the standard technique for clinical applications and standards for "susceptible" and "susceptible at increased dosage" and "resistant" are set by the European Committee on Antimicrobial Resistance (EUCAST) in the EU and CDC in the USA. The other method uses growth at step-wise doubling concentrations to determine the lowest concentration that prevents growth (Schuurmans et al. 2009). This method is more precise better reproducible, but also far more labor-intensive. The EU prescribes this method for the monitoring of AMR in implementing decision 2020/1729/EU to determine resistance in veterinary and foodborne microbes. Sime species of bacteria are intrinsically less sensitive or completely resistant to certain antimicrobials and there is considerable natural variation in the susceptibility. Therefore the distinction between susceptible and resistant is often subject to debate and hence standards are set by organisations such as EUCAST or CDC.

The term "One Health" is defined as the collaborative effort of multiple health science professions to attain optimal health for people, domestic animals, wildlife, plants, and our environment (McEwen and Collignon 2018). This approach recognizes the interdependent human, animal, and environmental dimensions of antimicrobial resistance. Governments worldwide and many intergovernmental agencies use the One Health approach to develop policies to address the problems posed by antimicrobial resistance, since it takes the complexity and ecological nature into account using a coordinated, multisectoral approach.

Development and Spreading of Resistance

Development and selection of resistance is regarded as the unavoidable consequence of usage of antimicrobials (Holmes et al. 2016). When microbes survive exposure to antibiotics, cellular adaptations resulting in resistance almost immediately occur (Handel et al. 2013). This implies that exposure to non-lethal concentrations of antibiotics forms a risk for development of resistance (Ter Kuile et al. 2016; Llewelyn et al. 2017). The perfect method for applying antibiotics consists of exposing the pathogens to a concentration high enough to kill all, and also high enough not to cause resistance in other microbes. In reality this is not possible, because there will always be gradients, and thus areas with non-lethal concentrations. In the veterinary practice, uneven distribution, spilling, or underdosing will cause differences in exposure and thus also low levels. In animals or in humans, the concentration changes with time, because after uptake into the bloodstream, drugs are excreted and break down. After some time, a new dose is applied, causing a new peak concentration and subsequent decline. A lower limit at which no selection for resistance takes place is defined for only very few drug/bug combinations. For those antibiotic, primarily beta-lactams and aminoglycosides, and bacteria combinations that have been investigated, the limit for no selection lies around 10% of the MIC (Andersson and Hughes 2014; Hughes 2014). In the case of fluoroquinolones, development of resistance already occurs at very low concentrations, at times less than 1% of the MIC (Gullberg et al. 2014).

The difference between bactericidal antibiotics, that kill bacteria and bacteriostatic compounds that reduce or stop the growth, is reflected in the development of resistance (Hasan et al. 2021). When bacteria survive exposure to antimicrobials, the develop resistance against bactericidal drug faster than against their bacteriostatic counterparts (van der Horst et al. 2011; Handel et al. 2014; Hoeksema et al. 2018). To survive exposure the concentrations the microbe is confronted with should by definition be below the MIC. During such exposure, the first changes in gene expression occur in less than 1 h and after a few hours the expression of between 100 and 200 genes, depending on the drug, is adapted (Zhou et al. 2011; Handel et al. 2013, 2014; Teichmann et al. 2024, 2025). These genes are often involved in metabolism. These changes at the expression levels cause increases of the MIC between 4 and 16 times, often already causing moderate clinical resistance. This has more practical consequences than would be expected at first, because an initial antibiotic treatment prescribed by a primary care physician can increase the MIC of a pathogen enough to make it resistant for all practical purposes against the applied antibiotic (Feng et al. 2014). After a few days at step-wise increasing, but non-lethal levels, DNA mutations start to occur that increase the MIC by factors between 100 and 10.000 (Handel et al. 2013; Hoeksema et al. 2019). This type of *de novo* development of resistance can occur for almost every drug-bug combination whenever there is exposure to non-lethal concentrations of antibiotics. There is no quantitative information on how large the role of this process is in development and spreading of resistance, but that it happens seems clear.

The role of plasmids in spreading resistance is better documented quantitatively (Davies and Davies 2010; Partridge et al. 2018). Since plasmids are multiplied independently of the chromosome, maintain themselves by toxin-antitoxin systems and are easily exchanged between microbes, they spread resistance on a large scale (Darphorn et al. 2021a, b, 2022). This process is indicated as "horizontal gene transfer" (HGT) (Tahmasebi et al. 2025). A large number of plasmids that have been described in the literature contain genes that code for antimicrobial resistance and for almost all antibiotics resistance genes are known (Aminov 2009; Darphorn et al. 2021a, b). Transfer of resistance plasmids occurs mostly between related bacterial species, but taxonomic relatedness is not required (Partridge et al. 2018). The presence of antibiotics in the environment hampers rather than stimulates the transfer of plasmids (Schuurmans et al. 2014; Handel et al. 2015). After transfer the resistance genes must be expressed to provide a selective advantage upon exposure to antibiotics (Munita and Arias 2016; Stepanenko and Heng 2017). Concentrations of antibiotics that do not kill the susceptible potential receptor cell, but do select for resistance form the greatest risk for HGT mediated spreading of resistance (Ter Kuile et al. 2016). Resistance plasmids can also cause co-selection, when resistance genes for two different antibiotics are located on the same plasmid (Kim et al. 2021). In such cases exposure to one antibiotic will also select resistance for the other.

Co-selection and transfer of resistance genes occur more often to plasmid bound resistance than in the case of resistance caused by chromosomal resistance genes or by chromosomal DNA mutations. An example is the spreading of plasmid bound ESBL types of resistance and the chromosomally encoded *ampC* gene mediated resistance. Because the ESBL genes are plasmid-bound, they transfer more easily and faster than the *ampC* gene. An in-between phenomenon is the amplification of DNA fragments around a resistance gene that at increased copy numbers causes more resistance and can also be transferred between cells (Darphorn et al. 2021a, b; Nong et al. 2024). As a result, plasmid encoded antimicrobial resistance is a bigger problem for public health than comparable resistance that is encoded by genes located on the chromosome.

It can be concluded from the discussion above that most important risk for both for *de novo* development of resistance and for transfer of plasmid mediated resistance is exposure to concentration of antibiotics below the MIC (Ter Kuile et al. 2016; Llewelyn et al. 2017). Exposure of bacteria in the veterinary sector to such concentrations is the unavoidable consequence of all other methods of application of antibiotics other than by injection. When antibiotics are dissolved in the drinking water, not all animals will get the same dose, and antibiotics can form deposits in the tubing and subsequently redissolve. When antibiotics are mixed in to the feed transfer between batches can occur and spreading drugs over the feed causes unequal distribution as well.

The State of Resistance in the EU

For the purpose of policy making concerning antimicrobial resistance, the state of affairs is continuously being monitored by governments worldwide both in human healthcare and in the agricultural sector (Antimicrobial Resistance 2022). In addition, universities and other research institutes investigate resistance against antibiotics in almost any environment (Baker et al. 2023). The microorganisms being monitored are usually the indicator organism *E. coli*, the pathogens of the genera *Salmonella* and *Campylobacter*. Sometimes the group of "*Enterobacteriaceae*" is included as well. The reports on this monitoring allow the analysis of trends over the years. Next, the situation in areas with differing antimicrobial policies can be compared. Below the situation in the EU will be analysed to create a picture of the state of resistance at the moment of writing.

Within the EU more antimicrobials are used for treating food-producing animals, almost 54,000 tons in 2021, than for human health care, just over 27,500 tons (EFSA/ECDC 2024a, b). In the EU the monitoring of resistance in the agricultural sector is regulated in the Commission Implementing Decision (EU) 2020/1729. Individual member states have their own reporting systems, but the EU prescribed data are always part of that. In 2024 the EU agencies EFSA and ECDC published the report "The European Union summary report on antimicrobial resistance in zoonotic and indicator bacteria from humans, animals and food in 2021–2022" (EFSA-ECDC 2024). The JIACRA reports of EFSA and ECDC analyses the usage of antibiotics for human health care and veterinary purposes. The fourth edition, reporting on the period 2019–2021 was published in 2024 as well (EFSA/ECDC 2024a, b). One example of member state reporting is the yearly MARAN series of The Netherlands, in which sales of antibiotics and the resistance monitoring data are reported (Veldman et al. 2023, 2024).

Each of these reports provides important information and significant insights. The JIACRA reports compare the resistance of human and veterinary isolates over the entire EU, enabling various correlations. Due to the completeness of the monitoring data within these reports, it is possible to compare human and agricultural and foodborne strains in a meaningful manner. Yearly reporting at more local level is very suitable for time course analysis discovering long-term trends and thereby discerning the effects of policy measures. The combination of the EFSA, JIACRA, and member state reporting can be used to draw conclusions that cannot be drawn based on the individual reports.

The Indicator Organism *E. coli*

The intestinal microbe *E. coli* is used as indicator organism to monitor the development and spreading of resistance, because it is found in all kinds of environments, on many animals and on foodstuffs (Poirel et al. 2018). Even though pathogenic *E. coli* strains exist, most isolates that are screened for resistance are harmless commensals. Hence, the indicator *E. coli* is not directly relevant for human health. Instead, it is used as gauge for overall antimicrobial resistance in the agricultural sector, which in the long-term may transfer to human health care. Many of the relevant resistance genes in *E. coli* are located on plasmids. Plasmid bound resistance is quantitatively more important for the spreading of resistance from the agricultural sector to human health care than resistant zoonoses (Hammerum et al. 2014; Loayza et al. 2020). The actual dispersion of resistance is mostly monitored using *E. coli* as indicator. In fact, it is not really an indicator since the role of *E. coli* in spreading resistance plasmids is larger than that of resistant pathogens (Zhang et al. 2020). Investigations concerning spreading of ESBL resistance focuses on "indicator" *E. coli*, because it is quantitatively the most important route (Aljohni et al. 2025). All in all, the common *E. coli* is considered more relevant for the general state of resistance than zoonotic species.

To ensure a valid comparison of the data from the member states, the prevalence of resistance is monitored in four categories of animals: slaughtered pigs, slaughtered meat calves younger than 1 year, broilers and turkeys. Because the sizes of the animal populations differ a "population correction unit" (PCU) is applied. Sales of antimicrobials are calculated by the European Medicines Agency (EMA) per PCU. To evaluate the overall state of resistance in the agricultural sector, a primary outcome indicator is used. This indicator is based on the percentage of E. coli that is sensitive to all antibiotics that are used in the testing panel. Hence it is an inverted indicator: the higher the number, the least resistance. Sample for slaughter pigs and meat calves are taken from the appendix. In addition, fresh pork and veal meat is sampled for ESBL *E. coli*. Similarly, broilers and turkeys are sampled. The measured resistance percentages vary greatly for the various drug-bug combinations, but some pathogens, such as Campylobacter, sometimes reach 100% for certain antibiotics, in this example fluoroquinolones (EFSA/ECDC 2024a, b). The same report states that over the EU as a whole the usage of antibiotics for food-producing animals was reduced by 44% between 2014 and 2021. Of these antibiotics belonging to the penicillins and tetracyclines are by far the most applied drugs, at just over and slightly less than 30% respectively.

The consequences of the usage on antimicrobials for development and spreading of resistance are analyzed in great detail with the use of statistics and multivariate analysis models in the JIACRA 4 report (EFSA/ECDC 2024a, b). Positive associations between usage for food-producing animals and resistance in bacteria isolated from these animals were shown for many antibiotics. In the cases that an association between usage and resistance in food-producing animals and resistance in human isolates could be demonstrated, it was most often resistance of the *E. coli* indicator that was statistically significant. For example, the association between tetracycline consumption of food-producing animals and resistance in human *Campylobacter coli* isolates was significant. In a different study the attribution of ESBL resistance in human isolates was analyzed in detail and between 20% and 25% turned out to be originally selected for in the agricultural sector (Mughini-Gras et al. 2019). When an antibiotic is not used at all for veterinary purposes due to legal restrictions, no resistance builds up in animals. This is demonstrated by the absence of meropenem resistance in animals and food related isolates (EFSA and ECDC 2020). A clear North-South gradient can be observed for multi-drug resistance, defined as resistance to antibiotics of at least three different classes, with far higher levels in the Southern EU member states than in the Northern counterparts In addition there is a correlation between the reduced usage of antibiotics in animals and an increase in the percentage of completely susceptible indicator *E. coli* in humans.

Veterinary application of antibiotics in The Netherlands can be used as example for the analysis of the effects of reducing antibiotic consumption. Yearly MARAN reports are available since 2000 on usage and resistance in the agricultural sector. In the year 2007 the minister of agriculture demanded a strong reduction of antimicrobial usage of the agricultural sector. Since that moment the overall usage is reduced by more than 70%. In the same period of time an average reduction of resistance percentage of around 50% can be discerned. There is a hysteresis of between 2 and 4 years for the resistance to actually go down after reduction of the amount of antibiotics used. EFSA concludes that not only the amount of antibiotics is relevant for resistance development, but also the way these are administered. Calves and pigs that are often treated individually have lower levels of resistant bacteria than broilers and turkeys that usually undergo group treatment (EFSA and ECDC 2020). Therefore, the conclusion can be drawn that the resistance reduction policies have been successful at reducing antimicrobial resistance, not only in animals but as a consequence also in human health care.

Salmonella

The various pathogenic species of the genus *Salmonella* remain a considerable burden on global; public health, not in the least because of widespread resistance to antimicrobials (Nazir et al. 2025). Overuse in livestock is a major contributor to selection and spreading of resistance. In the EU a wide range of resistance percentages were observed for tetracyclines, ampicillin and sulfonamides in food-producing animals and on meat with the exception of isolates from laying hens that had low resistance levels (EFSA/ECDC 2024a, b). Resistance to other beta-lactam antibiotics was relatively low in 2021 and 2022. In animals ESBL and AmpC driven resistance was low or very low, in humans very low. Overall resistance to third-generation cephalosporins was very low in human isolates, very low level in pigs and laying hens and low in broilers, turkeys and meat calves. No resistance to meropenem was reported in animals and only 5 cases (<0.1%) in humans. In general resistance to fluoroquinolones was high in most sectors and specifically very high for ciprofloxacin. Multidrug resistance was high at 30–40% depending on the serotype and the animals from which they were isolated. The mirror of that indicator, full susceptibility was between 30% and 70% depending on the same parameters. Analysis of the research conducted on horizontal gene transfer in Salmonella suggests that whole genome sequencing will be more than in the past the tool of choice for typing, monitoring and source attribution (Yan et al. 2024).

Campylobacter

Resistance levels of *Campylobacter coli* in livestock in the EU in the years 2021 and 2022 were higher than those of *C. jejuni*, when judged by complete susceptibility (EFSA/ECDC 2024a, b). Most data on *Campylobacter* are on isolates from poultry, fattening pigs and humans. Resistance in human isolates was intermediate between that of poultry, most resistant, and pigs that were least. These most recent EU data show only a direct correlation between fluoroquinolone resistance in pig *C. jejuni* isolates and those in humans. The same correlation was observed before as well (EFSA and ECDC 2020). The data over those years showed s stronger correlation between veterinary application of fluoroquinolones and resistance in human isolates than between human usage and resistance. For macrolides that same conclusion, better correlation between veterinary usage and human resistance than with human usage, had been reached before (ECDC et al. 2017). Over the years 2013 and 2014, but not 2015, a correlation between tetracycline usage for poultry and resistance in human isolates was found, but not between human usage and resistance. Given that the limited data all point in the same direction, usage for livestock correlates with resistance in human isolates, the implication is sufficiently serious to be a consideration in policymaking processes regarding the application of antimicrobials.

Specific Risks: ESBL, CPE, MRSA, Colistin and Panresistance

Several special forms of resistance that are encountered in livestock cause special problems for the human health care sector. Pathogens carrying these types of resistance are often indicated as "hospital bacteria" or "superbugs". Infections with these microbes and their subsequent spreading through health care facilities involve high costs for the stricken hospitals. Most of the time selection for this type of resistance occurs in the hospitals during necessary treatments of infections (Chokshi et al. 2019). In other cases, livestock can act as reservoir for resistance, such as extended spectrum beta-lactamase (ESBL)-carriers, carbapenemase producing Enterobacteriaceae (CPE), methicillin resistant Staphylococcus aureus (MRSA), and so-called panresistant bacteria. These are discussed below.

ESBLs

One form of resistance that is often discussed in the One Health framework is ESBL-carrying pathogens (Pana and Zaoutis 2018). ESBL carrying bacteria can destroy many antibiotics of the beta-lactam group, rendering hem ineffective for treatment. In addition to most penicillins, also monobactams and cephalosporins are demolished. The genes coding for ESBL's are often located on plasmids that can be rapidly transferred (Handel et al. 2015), as opposed to plasmids containing tetracycline resistance genes, that are transferred far slower (Schuurmans et al. 2014). In part because of the rapid interbacterial transfer ESBL-plasmids reach human health care from the veterinary sector. It is estimated that around 25% of the ESBL resistance in human health care is originally selected in the livestock sector (Mughini-Gras et al. 2019). Even more consequential is the model calculation that when the continuous supply of ESBL plasmids from agriculture is stopped, ESBL will slowly disappear from human health care. This suggests that reducing the ESBL form of resistance in the veterinary sector will have a much larger impact than the earlier mentioned 25% indicates. Since ESBL-bacteria are present throughout the environment livestock will repeatedly be exposed to these microbes (Martak et al. 2024). Manure plays a role in the transfer of ESBL's from agriculture to humans (Durso and Cook 2014). Therefore, better management of manure disposal and regulating streams of surface waters could reduce the exchange of ESBLs. Indeed, it turned out that dispersal of manure containing ESBL-carriers on fields just before a rain shower increased the ESBL concentrations in the surface waters surrounding these fields (Blaak et al. 2015). Otherwise, most reduction of ESBL transfer from livestock to humans is best prevented by reducing the selection at the root. This can be done by preventing the exposure of microbes to non-lethal concentrations, implemented by the principle "the highest dose the patient can handle, for the shortest time needed to clear the infection" (Ter Kuile et al. 2016; Llewelyn et al. 2017). In the case of pigs and calves, administering antibiotics by injection, rather than mixing them into the feed, will reduce the unneeded exposure to low levels of antibiotics considerably.

CPEs

Carbapenemase producing micro-organisms form a considerable risk for public health, since carbapenems are a means of last resort, much needed in hospitals when no other antibiotic is suitable (Somboro et al. 2018). CPE's are rarely encountered in livestock, only in a single sample in the EU in 2012 and 2022 (EFSA/ECDC 2024a, b). They have been found in samples of imported shrimps in The Netherlands (Veldman et al. 2019). The application of carbapenems for agricultural purposes is prohibited in the EU (regulation EU 2019/6). CPEs are, however, considered an emerging risk and in addition they are classified as priority pathogens (Macesic et al. 2025). As a result, the chances of carbapenem resistance being directly selected in the agricultural sector are minimal. CPEs are rarely resistant only to carbapenems. In fact, they are often multidrug resistant. What can happen is that CPEs are introduced to livestock, which is subsequently treated with an antibiotic that the CPE's are also resistant to.

In Germany CPEs were discovered on pigs that had never been treated with a carbapenem (Pulss et al. 2017; Irrgang et al. 2019). However, in later years no CPEs were found in an extensive survey of German pig farms (Effelsberg et al. 2021). Transfer of a carbapenem resistant *E. coli* from wild birds and insects to poultry has been demonstrated in China (Wang et al. 2017). In a wet market in Hong Kong, CPEs were found in samples derived from fish cultivated on fresh water and on pork (Sapugahawatte et al. 2020). If CPEs were to gain a foothold in livestock, the exposure to other antibiotics would be a permanent selective pressure, ensuring that the CPE's remain within flocks and herds. Migrating birds form a specific risk for the introduction of CPE's in livestock (Kock et al. 2018). In fact several groups of CPE containing strains exist, each with their own spreading pattern (van Duin and Doi 2017). A quantitative risk assessment predicting the livestock sector with the highest risk of CPE introduction, identified pig farms as being most at risk (Dankittipong et al. 2022). This prediction is in agreement with actual observations in the field (Pauly et al. 2020).

When considering measures to counter CPE in livestock there are several considerations. First of all, CPEs are often harmless commensals that do not cause disease in humans (Logan and Weinstein 2017; Madec et al. 2017). The carbapenem resistance only becomes a public health risk when the resistance is transferred to a pathogen, such as the ESKAPE species. Most of the time the source human-to human transfer, often related to foreign travel (van den Bunt et al. 2019; Kock et al. 2021). For that reason, imported foodstuffs cannot be rejected for carrying CPE's. Hence, it would also not be logical to take expensive countermeasures with a lot of impact on food production, such as clearing a complete farm, to eliminate this risk.

Still the risk that a small but non-negligible source of CPE in agriculture becomes a permanent cause of human infections cannot be ignored. Given the impact of a CPE outbreak within the human health care this risk requires continuous vigilance. An obligation to report CPE whenever encountered, both in the human health care and in other sectors would be instrumental for that aim.

MRSA

Methicillin resistant *Staphylococcus aureus* is endemic in many countries and causes considerable morbidity in hospitals and in the community. The livestock associated strain belonging to the clonal complex 398, often indicated as MRSA LA-398, is often encountered in pigs and chickens. Workers on infected farms often carry this strain, while workers on otherwise similar farms that are free from this pathogen, don't (Voss et al. 2005; Geenen et al. 2013). Despite the presence of MRSA CC398 and a comparable isolate mecC MRSA on livestock in the UK, only 4 out of 1242 human isolates that were classified belonged to the livestock associated categories (Paterson 2020). This suggest that these LA strains are not overly successful at infecting humans. However, in countries where the human carriage levels of MRSA are much lower, such as Denmark and The Netherlands, the contribution of the LA-MRSA strains to the overall human MRSA pool is roughly half (Sieber et al. 2018), or even more (de Greeff et al. 2019). Since the prevalence in The Netherlands was very low compared to the surrounding countries, 1.2%, the conclusion remains that LA-MRSA does not spread much in the human population. It is therefore only useful to take measures to reduce the presence of MRSA if the prevalence among humans and at farms is very low. Otherwise, the "search and destroy" policies that most hospitals in areas with low MRSA prevalence are far more effective.

Colistin

One of the means of last resort when a pathogen is resistant to all usual antimicrobials is colistin, also known as polymyxin A (de Greeff et al. 2019). Resistance against this antibiotic is therefore highly undesirable, even though it will not be used in large quantities for human medicine, due to its side effects. In the EU in 2021 0.7 mg colistin per kg biomass was used for humans, compared to 2.5 mg/kg for livestock (EFSA/ECDC 2024a, b). It is therefore particularly worrisome that plasmid-bound resistance against colistin is spreading (Liu et al. 2024). The European Antimicrobial Resistance Genes Surveillance Network (EURGen-Net) surveys colistin resistance within the EU. Over the period 2014–2021 there was a significant correlation between colistin usage and resistance in *E. coli* in isolates from chickens, but less so from pigs. Still levels of colistin suage were so low that statistical analysis was not always possible. Colistin resistance was very low in the Netherlands, but considerably higher in chickens in Germany, where it was used about 30 times more often for these animals (Veldman et al. 2019). Outside of the EU colistin is used more often for livestock, even though it is qualified as one of the highest priority critically important antimicrobials by the WHO (Gharaibeh and Shatnawi 2019). As reasoned above for carbapenemase producers, it is also not very useful to implement ultra strict measures for colistin resistance in the veterinary sector. The gain for public health is not enough to justify costly interventions.

Pan Resistance

Analysis of resistomes points out the increased risk of pan resistance for food chains, as microbiomes can be influenced in a negative manner (Yuan et al. 2024). Resistance against all classes of antibiotics remains rare in human health care, but does occur sporadically (Sieswerda et al. 2020). The spread via plasmids of genes coding for colistin resistance in E. coli cause sometimes pan resistance that coincides with increased virulence (Falgenhauer et al. 2017). Such strains that are resistant to all classes of antimicrobials seem to originate primarily from hospitals (Pecora et al. 2015). The contribution from the veterinary sector remains limited. Just as in the two cases discussed above, it is therefore not needed to already implement far going measures to counter pan resistance at the farm level. An ad-hoc risk assessment of an actual strain discovered at a farm may evaluate the risks for public health as very limited.

Microbiological Criteria

There are no separate laws and regulations for the resistant versions of microbes on foodstuffs, that would differ from the rules for their susceptible counterparts. At the moment the legal tools for countering high-risk resistant versions of bacteria for which there are no laws concerning the susceptible versions, are limited. In the case of foodstuffs this problem may be solved by formulating microbiological criteria for specific high-risk forms of resistance, such as carbapenemase production or pan resistance. In that case the competent authority will have the legal means to intervene when microbes with high-risk resistance are encountered. More and more taxonomy based on whole genome sequencing is being used as typing methodology for microbes. These WGS data can also be applied to identify resistance genes on isolates from foodstuffs (Frazao et al. 2020). After confirmation that the genotype indeed caused a resistant phenotype, the relevant law enforcement agency can take the appropriate measures.

Relationship Veterinary—Human

In the EU 38% of all antibiotics, measured in tons of active compounds, is used for humans and 62% for livestock (EFSA/ECDC 2024a, b), in agreement with earlier worldwide estimates (Cully 2014). That resistance selected for in the agricultural sector can subsequently end up in human health care is by now generally accepted. The large scale studies of EFSA and ECDC show that for some drug/bug combinations, the resistance in human isolates correlates more to veterinary usage than to usage of that particular antibiotic for humans (ECDC et al. 2017; EFSA/ECDC 2024a, b). One example is the observation that tetracycline resistance in human *Salmonella* isolates does not correlate with human tetracycline usage, but that there is a correlation between tetracycline resistance of livestock and human isolates. Tetracycline resistance in livestock does correlate to veterinary application of this drug, so in the end resistance in human isolates correlates with veterinary usage. A possible explanation may (Horvat and Kovacevic 2025) be that human usage is a fraction of the veterinary tetracycline application. Therefore, almost the entire selection pressure for tetracycline resistance originates in the veterinary sector. As a result, there is also no correlation between human tetracycline usage and resistance in human indicator *E. coli* isolates, but veterinary usage and resistance in livestock isolates do correlate with resistance in human isolates. Another observation supporting this notion is that when comparing resistance in several countries, resistance in human feces isolates was higher when the corresponding drug was allowed for veterinary purposes in that country (Forslund et al. 2013).

The data to make a quantitative overall attribution of resistance in human health care that was originally selected in livestock, is lacking (Pires et al. 2018; Hibbert et al. 2024). In the case of ESBL *E. coli* such attribution could only be established in a large study involving several countries (Mughini-Gras et al. 2019). Taking into account considerable margins of uncertainty, it seems that between 20% and 25% of the ESBL resistance encountered in human *E. coli* isolates originates from the agricultural sector. There are several pathways via which the ESBL genes ended up in the human E. coli isolates, the food chain being only one of these (Mughini-Gras et al. 2019). The correlation between veterinary usage and human health care resistance is much stronger in the case of tetracycline than for ESBL. This can be explained by the fact that tetracycline is mostly used for livestock and rarely for humans, while beta-lactams are used for both humans and animals (EFSA/ECDC 2024a, b).

Prevention of Development and Spreading of Resistance

All stakeholders involved in meat production support the overall aim of reducing the negative effects of livestock raising for human health care. This includes the selection of resistance. For a long time it was unclear how best to achieve this aim, because scientific information on the dose-response relationship was lacking. It was not clear how much usage of antibiotics and which manner of using caused how much resistance (Christaki et al. 2020). Recently, principles have been formulated for prudent use in the framework of a One Health approach (Horvat and Kovacevic 2025). These principles are translated in three main goals: (1) Reduce the total amount of antimicrobials used for livestock; (2) avoid development and spreading of resistance as much as possible by applying optimal methods for application. (3) Preserve important antibiotics for human health care for use in humans only.

In order to design cost-efficient measures for preventing and reducing resistance two factors need to be understood to some extent: (1) the driving factors for development and spreading of resistance and (2) the proportion of the resistance selected in the agricultural sector that is transferred to human health care. When patients are infected by a resistant variant of a pathogen, costs of therapy are higher, both in patient suffering and in financial terms. For every measure that is taken in the veterinary practice to cost of the measure at the farm should be compared to the gains for human health care. The implementation of a proposed measure can then be decided upon based on usefulness and necessity. The global burden of antimicrobial resistance is estimated as just over a million deaths per year attributable to AMR and around five million associated with it (Antimicrobial Resistance 2022). The financial costs for the EU are estimated at 1.5 billion Euro per year (EU 2017; Cassini et al. 2019b). This may seem like an enormous amount of money, but, if about one quarter of these cost are to be attributed to veterinary practice, the amount farms are responsible for become around 400 million Euros. Forcing all European farms to implement expensive measures is likely to be more costly than that. Hence countermeasures at the farm level should be carefully considered also from a financial point of view. When doing so, the possibility that not taking a certain measure might contribute to uncontrollable spreading of resistance, with all costs associated to that, must also be weighed.

Reducing the Need for Antibiotic Usage

Obviously, the best way to counter development and spread of antimicrobial resistance is to eliminate the necessity of their application. Completely eliminating this need is an illusion, but important reductions can be achieved by measures at farms to prevent infections. This can be done by improved hygiene, better quality feed, vaccination when possible and improved farm management in general. Exchange of bacteria and exposure to resistant pathogens causes spreading of resistance (Collignon and McEwen 2019). Clean farms improve animal health and welfare (Van der Meer 2017), because dirt in the stables, sheds and barns causes infections, that subsequently reduce growth (Strauch 1991). Poor hygiene in the shed is a known cause of mastitis in milk cows (Visser et al. 2015). One important aspect of farm hygiene is therefore the absence of pathogenic microorganisms. These are not only present in dung, but also in other dirt of animal origin. Rats that feed on dirt also bring pathogens along. The costs of cleaning can be lowered by taking hygiene into account while designing and building a animal facility. For example: vertical surfaces that are easily washable, avoiding unneeded ledges, putting beams in such a way that they can be easily cleaned or don't accumulate dirt. These measures will also have a positive influence on farm economics, as revenues will go up and the costs for veterinary care will go down.

The microbiological quality of feed directly influences animal health (Davies et al. 2004; Kaur et al. 2023). The various *Salmonella* strains are mostly introduced at farms through the feed, after which the animals are re-infected through the manure (Wilhelm et al. 2012). At the moment of writing there are no rules, regulations or microbiological criteria regarding the microbiological quality of feed. As a start it might be useful to monitor the microbiological quality of feed, in order to be a able to assess whether improving feed quality could indeed positively influence animal health by reducing exposure to *Salmonella* and possibly other pathogens. In contrast to *Salmonella*, the occurrence of *Campylobacter* on livestock correlates more bad hygiene in the living quarters than with bad quality feed (Nather et al. 2009).

In the case of animals held in closed living quarters, such as stables, sheds and barns, most antibiotics are used to fight airway infections. The chance of pulmonary disease is increased by exposure of the lungs to pathogens, which is in turn caused by bad air quality due to poor ventilation (Roland et al. 2016). Livestock housing, whether for chickens, pigs or cows, is often equipped with automatic ventilation. For the prevention of pulmonary diseases in the animals, good functioning of such systems is essential. This requires constant monitoring of air quality and accurate control of the equipment, so that the air is clean. This way airway infections can be prevented (Roland et al. 2016). Research into the relationship between air quality and animal health is needed to formulate microbiological standards for the air quality in livestock holding facilities.

Methods for Administering Antimicrobials

Compared to milking cow meat calves are much more often treated with antibiotics (Veldman et al. 2019, 2024). One of the reasons for this difference is that they are often transported at a very young age between their place of birth and the place where they will be grown to their slaughter weight (Renaud and Pardon 2022). Since they are brought together with similar calves for many other locations, they exchange pathogens, increasing the chance of infections (Marcato et al. 2018). Young calves have an underdeveloped immune system and are therefore more sensitive to infections than older animals (Siddiqui et al. 2012). Hence, when immunologically immature calves are collected form several locations, an increased use of antibiotics seems unavoidable. Similarly, piglets are also often treated with antibiotics shortly after weaning. In these situations, treatment is usually applied to whole groups.

In the past group treatment was almost always provided by mixing antibiotics through the feed or the drinking water. Healthy animals eat and drink more than sick and consequently take in higher doses of the medicine. Dissolving antibiotics in the drinking water leads to deposition in the tubes with redissolving afterwards. Another method was "topdressing": distributing the antibiotics over the feed. This method causes a very uneven distribution of the drugs, so the animals would get vastly differing amounts (Alleweldt 2010). For almost all animals other than chickens, the optimal manner of applying antimicrobials is by injection. All animals will get the correct dose, there is no spillage, or leftovers in the feed, and the microbiota of the intestines are less exposed to antibiotics than when these are mixed in the feed or water.

Challenges Regarding Treatment of Infections in Livestock

Animal health and welfare requires that veterinarians have the possibility to treat bacterial infections in livestock with antimicrobials. It is not even certain that a complete ban on the usage of antibiotics for livestock would reduce the overall resistance, because animals would become a reservoir of bacteria, many of which would be resistant as a result of exposure to antibiotics outside of the agricultural sector. The challenge is to achieve optimal animal health at minimal costs, in the sense of resistance selected for and increased costs for human public health. Exactly that question is addressed in the following chapters of this book. The following main topics are addressed: Which measures can be taken to prevent unnecessary veterinary usage of antimicrobials? What are the consequences of antimicrobials from farms ending up in the environment? After selection has taken place on farms, how can spreading be prevented?

References

Aljohni MS, Harun-Ur-Rashid M, Selim S (2025) Emerging threats: antimicrobial resistance in extended-spectrum beta-lactamase and carbapenem-resistant Escherichia coli. Microb Pathog 200:107275

Alleweldt F (2010) Evaluation of the EU legislative framework in the field of medicated feed. FCEC, Brussels, p 188

Aminov RI (2009) The role of antibiotics and antibiotic resistance in nature. Environ Microbiol 11:2970–2988

Andersson DI, Hughes D (2014) Microbiological effects of sublethal levels of antibiotics. Nat Rev Microbiol 12:465–478

Antimicrobial Resistance Collaborators (2022) Global burden of bacterial antimicrobial resistance in 2019: a systematic analysis. Lancet 399:629–655

Baker KS, Jauneikaite E, Hopkins KL et al (2023) Genomics for public health and international surveillance of antimicrobial resistance. Lancet Microbe 4:e1047–e1055

Berdy J (2012) Thoughts and facts about antibiotics: where we are now and where we are heading. J Antibiot (Tokyo) 65:385–395

Blaak H, Lynch G, Italiaander R, Hamidjaja RA, Schets FM, de Roda Husman AM (2015) Multidrug-resistant and extended spectrum beta-lactamase-producing Escherichia coli in Dutch surface water and wastewater. PLoS One 10:e0127752

Cassini A, Plachouras D, Monnet DL (2019a) Attributable deaths caused by infections with antibiotic-resistant bacteria in France—Authors' reply. Lancet Infect Dis 19:129–130

Cassini A, Hogberg LD, Plachouras D et al (2019b) Attributable deaths and disability-adjusted life-years caused by infections with antibiotic-resistant bacteria in the EU and the European Economic Area in 2015: a population-level modelling analysis. Lancet Infect Dis 19:56–66

Chatterjee A, Modarai M, Naylor NR, Boyd SE, Atun R, Barlow J, Holmes AH, Johnson A, Robotham JV (2018) Quantifying drivers of antibiotic resistance in humans: a systematic review. Lancet Infect Dis 18:e368–e378

Chokshi A, Sifri Z, Cennimo D, Horng H (2019) Global contributors to antibiotic resistance. J Glob Infect Dis 11:36–42

Christaki E, Marcou M, Tofarides A (2020) Antimicrobial resistance in bacteria: mechanisms, evolution, and persistence. J Mol Evol 88:26–40

Collignon PJ, McEwen SA (2019) One Health–Its importance in helping to better control antimicrobial resistance. Trop Med Infect Dis 4(1):22

Cully M (2014) Public health: the politics of antibiotics. Nature 509:S16–S17

Dankittipong N, Fischer EAJ, Swanenburg M, Wagenaar JA, Stegeman AJ, de Vos CJ (2022) Quantitative risk assessment for the introduction of Carbapenem-Resistant Enterobacteriaceae (CPE) into Dutch livestock farms. Antibiotics (Basel) 11(2):281

Darphorn TS, Bel K, Koenders-van Sint Anneland BB, Brul S, Ter Kuile BH (2021a) Antibiotic resistance plasmid composition and architecture in Escherichia coli isolates from meat. Sci Rep 11:2136

Darphorn TS, Hu Y, Koenders-van Sintanneland BB, Brul S, Ter Kuile BH (2021b) Multiplication of ampC upon exposure to a beta-lactam antibiotic results in a transferable transposon in Escherichia coli. Int J Mol Sci 22(17):9230

Darphorn TS, Koenders-van Sintanneland BB, Grootemaat AE, van der Wel NN, Brul S, Ter Kuile BH (2022) Transfer dynamics of multi-resistance plasmids in Escherichia coli isolated from meat. PLoS One 17:e0270205

Davies J, Davies D (2010) Origins and evolution of antibiotic resistance. Microbiol Mol Biol Rev 74:417–433

Davies PR, Scott Hurd H, Funk JA, Fedorka-Cray PJ, Jones FT (2004) The role of contaminated feed in the epidemiology and control of Salmonella enterica in pork production. Foodborne Pathog Dis 1:202–215

de Greeff SC, Mouton JW, Schoffelen AF, Verduin CM (2019) NethMap 2019 consumption of antimicrobial agents and antimicrobial resistance among medically important bacteria in The Netherlands. RIVM, Bilthoven, p 166

Dunachie SJ, Day NP, Dolecek C (2020) The challenges of estimating the human global burden of disease of antimicrobial resistant bacteria. Curr Opin Microbiol 57:95–101

Durso LM, Cook KL (2014) Impacts of antibiotic use in agriculture: what are the benefits and risks? Curr Opin Microbiol 19:37–44

ECDC, EFSA & EMA (2017) ECDC/EFSA/EMA second joint report on the integrated analysis of the consumption of antimicrobial agents and occurrence of antimicrobial resistance in bacteria from humans and food-producing animals—Joint Interagency Antimicrobial Consumption and Resistance Analysis (JIACRA) Report. EFSA J 15:135

Effelsberg N, Kobusch I, Linnemann S, Hofmann F, Schollenbruch H, Mellmann A, Boelhauve M, Kock R, Cuny C (2021) Prevalence and zoonotic transmission of colistin-resistant and carbapenemase-producing Enterobacterales on German pig farms. One Health 13:100354

EFSA & ECDC (2020) The European Union summary report on antimicrobial resistance in zoonotic and indicator bacteria from humans, animals and food in 2017/2018. EFSA J 18:166

EFSA/ECDC (2024a) The European Union summary report on antimicrobial resistance in zoonotic and indicator bacteria from humans, animals and food in 2021–2022. EFSA J 21(3):e07867
EFSA/ECDC (2024b) JIACRA 4 Antimicrobial consumption and resistance in bacteria from humans and food-producing animals. EFSA J 172
EFSA-ECDC (2024) The European Union summary report on antimicrobial resistance in zoonotic and indicator bacteria from humans, animals and food in 2021–2022. EFSA J 22(2):e8583
EU (2017) A European one health action plan against antimicrobial resistance (AMR). European Commission, Brussels
Falgenhauer L, Ghosh H, Doijad S et al (2017) Genome analysis of the Carbapenem- and Colistin-resistant Escherichia coli isolate NRZ14408 reveals horizontal gene transfer pathways towards panresistance and enhanced virulence. Antimicrob Agents Chemother 61(4):e02359–e02316
Feng Y, Handel N, de Groot MH, Brul S, Schultsz C, Ter Kuile BH (2014) Experimental simulation of the effects of an initial antibiotic treatment on a subsequent treatment after initial therapy failure. Antibiotics 3:49–63
Forslund K, Sunagawa S, Kultima JR, Mende DR, Arumugam M, Typas A, Bork P (2013) Country-specific antibiotic use practices impact the human gut resistome. Genome Res 23:1163–1169
Frazao MR, Cao G, Medeiros MIC, Duque SDS, Allard MW, Falcao JP (2020) Antimicrobial Resistance profiles and phylogenetic analysis of Campylobacter jejuni strains isolated in Brazil by whole genome sequencing. Microb Drug Resist 27:660–669
Freitas AR, Karpinski TM, Li B (2020) Editorial: antimicrobials and anticancers of bacterial origins. Front Microbiol 11:842
Geenen PL, Graat EA, Haenen A, Hengeveld PD, Van Hoek AH, Huijsdens XW, Kappert CC, Lammers GA, Van Duijkeren E, Van De Giessen AW (2013) Prevalence of livestock-associated MRSA on Dutch broiler farms and in people living and/or working on these farms. Epidemiol Infect 141:1099–1108
Gharaibeh MH, Shatnawi SQ (2019) An overview of colistin resistance, mobilized colistin resistance genes dissemination, global responses, and the alternatives to colistin: a review. Vet World 12:1735–1746
Gullberg E, Albrecht LM, Karlsson C, Sandegren L, Andersson DI (2014) Selection of a multidrug resistance plasmid by sublethal levels of antibiotics and heavy metals. MBio 5:e01918–e01914
Hammerum AM, Larsen J, Andersen VD et al (2014) Characterization of extended-spectrum beta-lactamase (ESBL)-producing Escherichia coli obtained from Danish pigs, pig farmers and their families from farms with high or no consumption of third- or fourth-generation cephalosporins. J Antimicrob Chemother 69:2650–2657
Handel N, Schuurmans JM, Brul S, Ter Kuile BH (2013) Compensation of the metabolic costs of antibiotic resistance by physiological adaptation in Escherichia coli. Antimicrob Agents Chemother 57:3752–3762
Handel N, Schuurmans JM, Feng Y, Brul S, Ter Kuile BH (2014) Interaction between mutations and regulation of gene expression during development of de novo antibiotic resistance. Antimicrob Agents Chemother 58:4371–4379
Handel N, Otte S, Jonker M, Brul S, ter Kuile BH (2015) Factors that affect transfer of the IncI1 beta-lactam resistance plasmid pESBL-283 between E. coli strains. PLoS One 10:e0123039
Hasan CM, Dutta D, Nguyen ANT (2021) Revisiting antibiotic resistance: mechanistic foundations to evolutionary outlook. Antibiotics (Basel) 11(1):40
Hibbert T, Krpetic Z, Latimer J, Leighton H, McHugh R, Pottenger S, Wragg C, James CE (2024) Antimicrobials: an update on new strategies to diversify treatment for bacterial infections. Adv Microb Physiol 84:135–241
Ho CS, Wong CTH, Aung TT et al (2025) Antimicrobial resistance: a concise update. Lancet Microbe 6:100947
Hoeksema M, Brul S, Ter Kuile BH (2018) Influence of reactive oxygen species on de novo acquisition of resistance to bactericidal antibiotics. Antimicrob Agents Chemother 62(6):e02354–e02317

Hoeksema M, Jonker MJ, Brul S, Ter Kuile BH (2019) Effects of a previously selected antibiotic resistance on mutations acquired during development of a second resistance in Escherichia coli. BMC Genomics 20:284

Holmes AH, Moore LS, Sundsfjord A, Steinbakk M, Regmi S, Karkey A, Guerin PJ, Piddock LJ (2016) Understanding the mechanisms and drivers of antimicrobial resistance. Lancet 387:176–187

Horvat O, Kovacevic Z (2025) Human and veterinary medicine collaboration: synergistic approach to address antimicrobial resistance through the lens of planetary health. Antibiotics (Basel) 14(1):38

Huebner C, Flessa S, Huebner NO (2019) The economic impact of antimicrobial stewardship programmes in hospitals: a systematic literature review. J Hosp Infect 102:369–376

Hughes D (2014) Selection and evolution of resistance to antimicrobial drugs. IUBMB Life 66:521–529

Irrgang A, Tenhagen BA, Pauly N, Schmoger S, Kaesbohrer A, Hammerl JA (2019) Characterization of VIM-1-Producing E. coli isolated from a German fattening pig farm by an improved isolation procedure. Front Microbiol 10:2256

Jorgensen JH, Ferraro MJ (2009) Antimicrobial susceptibility testing: a review of general principles and contemporary practices. Clin Infect Dis 49:1749–1755

Kaur H, Kaur G, Gupta T, Mittal D, Ali SA (2023) Integrating omics technologies for a comprehensive understanding of the microbiome and its impact on cattle production. Biology (Basel) 12(9):1200

Kim M, Park J, Kang M, Yang J, Park W (2021) Gain and loss of antibiotic resistant genes in multidrug resistant bacteria: One Health perspective. J Microbiol 59:535–545

Kock R, Daniels-Haardt I, Becker K, Mellmann A, Friedrich AW, Mevius D, Schwarz S, Jurke A (2018) Carbapenem-resistant Enterobacteriaceae in wildlife, food-producing, and companion animals: a systematic review. Clin Microbiol Infect 24:1241–1250

Kock R, Herr C, Kreienbrock L, Schwarz S, Tenhagen BA, Walther B (2021) Multiresistant gram-negative pathogens – a zoonotic problem. Dtsch Arztebl Int 118:579–589

Lhermie G, Tauer LW, Grohn YT (2018a) An assessment of the economic costs to the U.S. dairy market of antimicrobial use restrictions. Prev Vet Med 160:63–67

Lhermie G, Tauer LW, Grohn YT (2018b) The farm cost of decreasing antimicrobial use in dairy production. PLoS One 13:e0194832

Lima LM, Silva B, Barbosa G, Barreiro EJ (2020) beta-lactam antibiotics: an overview from a medicinal chemistry perspective. Eur J Med Chem 208:112829

Liu JH, Liu YY, Shen YB, Yang J, Walsh TR, Wang Y, Shen J (2024) Plasmid-mediated colistin-resistance genes: mcr. Trends Microbiol 32:365–378

Llewelyn MJ, Fitzpatrick JM, Darwin E, Sarah Tonkin C, Gorton C, Paul J, Peto TEA, Yardley L, Hopkins S, Walker AS (2017) The antibiotic course has had its day. BMJ 358:j3418

Loayza F, Graham JP, Trueba G (2020) Factors obscuring the role of E. coli from domestic animals in the global antimicrobial resistance crisis: an evidence-based review. Int J Environ Res Public Health 17(9):3061

Logan LK, Weinstein RA (2017) The epidemiology of carbapenem-resistant Enterobacteriaceae: the impact and evolution of a global menace. J Infect Dis 215:S28–S36

Macesic N, Uhlemann AC, Peleg AY (2025) Multidrug-resistant Gram-negative bacterial infections. Lancet 405:257–272

Madec JY, Haenni M, Nordmann P, Poirel L (2017) Extended-spectrum beta-lactamase/AmpC- and carbapenemase-producing Enterobacteriaceae in animals: a threat for humans? Clin Microbiol Infect 23:826–833

Marcato F, van den Brand H, Kemp B, van Reenen K (2018) Evaluating potential biomarkers of health and performance in veal calves. Front Vet Sci 5:133

Martak D, Henriot CP, Hocquet D (2024) Environment, animals, and food as reservoirs of antibiotic-resistant bacteria for humans: One health or more? Infect Dis Now 54:104895

Maurya AP, Rajkumari J, Bhattacharjee A, Pandey P (2020) Development, spread and persistence of antibiotic resistance genes (ARGs) in the soil microbiomes through co-selection. Rev Environ Health 35:371–378

McEwen SA, Collignon PJ (2018) Antimicrobial Resistance: a one health perspective. Microbiol Spectr 6:521–547

Mughini-Gras L, Dorado-Garcia A, van Duijkeren E et al (2019) Attributable sources of community-acquired carriage of Escherichia coli containing beta-lactam antibiotic resistance genes: a population-based modelling study. Lancet Planet Health 3:e357–e369

Munita JM, Arias CA (2016) Mechanisms of Antibiotic Resistance. Microbiol Spectr 4(2):481–511

Mustafa AS (2024) Whole genome sequencing: applications in clinical bacteriology. Med Princ Pract 33:185–197

Nather G, Alter T, Martin A, Ellerbroek L (2009) Analysis of risk factors for Campylobacter species infection in broiler flocks. Poult Sci 88:1299–1305

Nazir J, Manzoor T, Saleem A, Gani U, Bhat SS, Khan S, Haq Z, Jha P, Ahmad SM (2025) Combatting Salmonella: a focus on antimicrobial resistance and the need for effective vaccination. BMC Infect Dis 25:84

Nong L, Jonker M, de Leeuw W, Wortel MT, Ter Kuile B (2024) Progression of ampC amplification during de novo amoxicillin resistance development in E. coli. mBio 16(2):e0298224

Pana ZD, Zaoutis T (2018) Treatment of extended-spectrum beta-lactamase-producing Enterobacteriaceae (ESBLs) infections: what have we learned until now? F1000Res 7:F1000

Partridge SR, Kwong SM, Firth N, Jensen SO (2018) Mobile genetic elements associated with antimicrobial resistance. Clin Microbiol Rev 31(4):e00088–e00017

Paterson GK (2020) Low prevalence of livestock-associated methicillin-resistant Staphylococcus aureus clonal complex 398 and mecC MRSA among human isolates in North-West England. J Appl Microbiol 128:1785–1792

Pauly N, Hammerl JA, Grobbel M, Kasbohrer A, Tenhagen BA, Malorny B, Schwarz S, Meemken D, Irrgang A (2020) Identification of a bla(VIM-1)-Carrying IncA/C(2) multiresistance plasmid in an Escherichia coli isolate recovered from the German food chain. Microorganisms 9(1):29

Pecora ND, Li N, Allard M, Li C, Albano E, Delaney M, Dubois A, Onderdonk AB, Bry L (2015) Genomically informed surveillance for carbapenem-resistant Enterobacteriaceae in a health care system. MBio 6:e01030

Pires SM, Duarte AS, Hald T (2018) Source attribution and risk assessment of antimicrobial resistance. Microbiol Spectr 6(3):619–635

Poirel L, Madec JY, Lupo A, Schink AK, Kieffer N, Nordmann P, Schwarz S (2018) Antimicrobial resistance in Escherichia coli. Microbiol Spectr 6:10–1128

Pulss S, Semmler T, Prenger-Berninghoff E, Bauerfeind R, Ewers C (2017) First report of an Escherichia coli strain from swine carrying an OXA-181 carbapenemase and the colistin resistance determinant MCR-1. Int J Antimicrob Agents 50:232–236

Qi W, Jonker MJ, de Leeuw W, Brul S, Ter Kuile BH (2023a) Reactive oxygen species accelerate de novo acquisition of antibiotic resistance in E. coli. iScience 26:108373

Qi W, Jonker MJ, Teichmann L, Wortel M, Ter Kuile BH (2023b) The influence of oxygen and oxidative stress on de novo acquisition of antibiotic resistance in E. coli and Lactobacillus lactis. BMC Microbiol 23:279

Renaud D, Pardon B (2022) Preparing male dairy calves for the veal and dairy beef industry. Vet Clin North Am Food Anim Pract 38:77–92

Roland L, Drillich M, Klein-Jobstl D, Iwersen M (2016) Invited review: influence of climatic conditions on the development, performance, and health of calves. J Dairy Sci 99:2438–2452

Sapugahawatte DN, Li C, Zhu C, Dharmaratne P, Wong KT, Lo N, Ip M (2020) Prevalence and characteristics of extended-spectrum-beta-lactamase-producing and carbapenemase-producing Enterobacteriaceae from freshwater fish and pork in wet markets of Hong Kong. mSphere 5(2):e00107–e00120

Schuurmans JM, Nuri Hayali AS, Koenders BB, ter Kuile BH (2009) Variations in MIC value caused by differences in experimental protocol. J Microbiol Methods 79:44–47

Schuurmans JM, van Hijum SA, Piet JR, Handel N, Smelt J, Brul S, ter Kuile BH (2014) Effect of growth rate and selection pressure on rates of transfer of an antibiotic resistance plasmid between E. coli strains. Plasmid 72:1–8

Siddiqui N, Price S, Hope J (2012) BCG vaccination of neonatal calves: potential roles for innate immune cells in the induction of protective immunity. Comp Immunol Microbiol Infect Dis 35:219–226

Sieber RN, Skov RL, Nielsen J, Schulz J, Price LB, Aarestrup FM, Larsen AR, Stegger M, Larsen J (2018) Drivers and dynamics of methicillin-resistant livestock-associated Staphylococcus aureus CC398 in pigs and humans in Denmark. mBio 9(6):e02142–e02118

Sieswerda E, van den Brand M, van den Berg RB, Strater J, Schouls L, van Dijk K, Budding AE (2020) Successful rescue treatment of sepsis due to a pandrug-resistant, NDM-producing Klebsiella pneumoniae using aztreonam powder for nebulizer solution as intravenous therapy in combination with ceftazidime/avibactam. J Antimicrob Chemother 75:773–775

Somboro AM, Osei Sekyere J, Amoako DG, Essack SY, Bester LA (2018) Diversity and proliferation of metallo-beta-lactamases: a clarion call for clinically effective metallo-beta-lactamase inhibitors. Appl Environ Microbiol 84(18):e00698–e00618

Stepanenko AA, Heng HH (2017) Transient and stable vector transfection: pitfalls, off-target effects, artifacts. Mutat Res 773:91–103

Strauch D (1991) Survival of pathogenic micro-organisms and parasites in excreta, manure and sewage sludge. Rev Sci Tech 10:813–846

Tahmasebi H, Arjmand N, Monemi M, Babaeizad A, Alibabaei F, Alibabaei N, Bahar A, Oksenych V, Eslami M (2025) From cure to crisis: understanding the evolution of antibiotic-resistant bacteria in human microbiota. Biomolecules 15(1):93

Teichmann L, Pasman R, Luitwieler S, Varriale C, Bengtsson-Palme J, Ter Kuile B (2024) Adaptation of Escherichia coli to ciprofloxacin and enrofloxacin: differential proteomics of the SOS response and RecA-independent mechanisms. Int J Antimicrob Agents 65:107420

Teichmann L, Luitwieler S, Bengtsson-Palme J, Ter Kuile B (2025) Fluoroquinolone-specific resistance trajectories in E. coli and their dependence on the SOS-response. BMC Microbiol 25:37

Ter Kuile BH, Kraupner N, Brul S (2016) The risk of low concentrations of antibiotics in agriculture for resistance in human health care. FEMS Microbiol Lett 363(19):fnw210

van den Bunt G, van Pelt W, Hidalgo L, Scharringa J, de Greeff SC, Schurch AC, Mughini-Gras L, Bonten MJM, Fluit AC (2019) Prevalence, risk factors and genetic characterisation of extended-spectrum beta-lactamase and carbapenemase-producing Enterobacteriaceae (ESBL-E and CPE): a community-based cross-sectional study, the Netherlands, 2014 to 2016. Euro Surveill 24(41):1800594

van der Horst MA, Schuurmans JM, Smid MC, Koenders BB, Ter Kuile BH (2011) De Novo acquisition of resistance to three antibiotics by Escherichia coli. Microb Drug Resist 17:141–147

Van der Meer Y (2017) Nutrition of pigs kept under low and high sanitary conditions: effects on amino acid and energy metabolism and damaging behaviour. WUR, Wageningen, p 182

van Duin D, Doi Y (2017) The global epidemiology of carbapenemase-producing Enterobacteriaceae. Virulence 8:460–469

Veldman KT, Mevius DJ, Wit B, Van Pelt W, Franz E, Heederik D (2019) MARAN 2019 monitoring of antimicrobial resistance and antibiotic usage in animals in the Netherlands in 2018. Wageningen Bioveterinary Research, Lelystad, p 82

Veldman KT, Wit B, Franz E, Heederik DJJ (2023) Monitoring of antimicrobial resistance and antibiotic usage in animals in the Netherlands in 2022. Wageningen Bioveterinary Research (WBVR), Lelystad, p 76

Veldman KT, Wit B, Franz E, Heederik DJJ (2024) Maran 2024 monitoring of antimicrobial resistance and antibiotic usage in animals in the Netherlands in 2023. Wageningen Bioveterinary Research, Wageningen, p 77

Visser K, Rommers J, Ipema B, Verkaik J, Gerritzen M, Van Reenen K (2015) Risicoanalyse dierenwelzijn zuivelketen. Wageningen UR Livestock Research, Wageningen, p 78

Voss A, Loeffen F, Bakker J, Klaassen C, Wulf M (2005) Methicillin-resistant Staphylococcus aureus in pig farming. Emerg Infect Dis 11:1965–1966

Walsh F, Duffy B (2013) The culturable soil antibiotic resistome: a community of multi-drug resistant bacteria. PLoS One 8:e65567

Wang Y, Zhang R, Li J et al (2017) Comprehensive resistome analysis reveals the prevalence of NDM and MCR-1 in Chinese poultry production. Nat Microbiol 2:16260

Wilhelm B, Rajic A, Parker S, Waddell L, Sanchez J, Fazil A, Wilkins W, McEwen SA (2012) Assessment of the efficacy and quality of evidence for five on-farm interventions for Salmonella reduction in grow-finish swine: a systematic review and meta-analysis. Prev Vet Med 107:1–20

Yan J, Doublet B, Wiedemann A (2024) Trends in horizontal gene transfer research in Salmonella antimicrobial resistance: a bibliometric analysis. Front Microbiol 15:1439664

Yuan M, Huang Z, Malakar PK, Pan Y, Zhao Y, Zhang Z (2024) Antimicrobial resistomes in food chain microbiomes. Crit Rev Food Sci Nutr 64:6953–6974

Zhang S, Abbas M, Rehman MU, Huang Y, Zhou R, Gong S, Yang H, Chen S, Wang M, Cheng A (2020) Dissemination of antibiotic resistance genes (ARGs) via integrons in Escherichia coli: a risk to human health. Environ Pollut 266:115260

Zhou K, Zhou L, Lim Q, Zou R, Stephanopoulos G, Too HP (2011) Novel reference genes for quantifying transcriptional responses of Escherichia coli to protein overexpression by quantitative PCR. BMC Mol Biol 12:18

Chapter 2
Preventive Measures to Minimise Veterinary Antibiotic Use and Their Impact on Antibiotic Resistance

Kees Veldman, Anita Dame-Korevaar, David Speksnijder, Zorana Kovačević, Roberto La Ragione, Aisling Glennie, Birgitta Duim, Luís Pedro Carmo, Katharina D. C. Stärk, and Benno ter Kuile

Abstract Interventions reducing antimicrobial usage in animals are associated with decreased antimicrobial resistance in animals and to a lesser extent to decreased antimicrobial resistance in humans. To prevent development and spread of antimicrobial resistance in farm animals, good farm management, infection prevention and prudent use of antimicrobials seem important focus points. Sensor-based techniques using artificial intelligence can improve farm management and monitoring of animals disease supporting prudent use of antimicrobials. To date, alternatives for antimicrobials have not shown efficacy comparable to curative antibiotic treatments, but more research is essential to explore the potential of using prebiotics, probiotics and postbiotics or other alternatives for antimicrobials treatments.

K. Veldman (✉) · A. Dame-Korevaar
Wageningen Bioveterinary Research, Lelystad, The Netherlands
e-mail: kees.veldman@wur.nl; anita.dame@wur.nl

D. Speksnijder · B. Duim
Faculty of Veterinary Medicine, University of Utrecht, Utrecht, The Netherlands
e-mail: D.C.Speksnijder@uu.nl; B.Duim@uu.nl

Z. Kovačević
Department of Veterinary Medicine, University of Novi Sad, Novi Sad, Serbia
e-mail: zorana.kovacevic@polj.edu.rs

R. La Ragione
School of Veterinary Medicine, and School of Biosciences, University of Surrey, Guildford, UK
e-mail: r.laragione@surrey.ac.uk

A. Glennie
Veterinary Medicines Directorate VMD, Addlestone, UK

Department for Environment, Food & Rural Affairs, London, UK
e-mail: a.glennie@vmd.gov.uk

B. ter Kuile (ed.), *Antimicrobial Resistance and Antibiotics Usage in Livestock*,
https://doi.org/10.1007/978-3-032-04598-0_2

In theory, these measures will jointly support further reduction of antimicrobial use in farm animals. However, the effectiveness also depends on the behavior of farmers and veterinarians. In a time of the rising awareness to fight antimicrobial resistance there is a strong need to rethink current livestock production systems comprehensively in the light of animal welfare and health, environmental implications, antimicrobial use and resistance and economic profitability for farmers. This goes beyond the individual farm level and requires a strong system thinking approach with input from a wide variety of scientific disciplines.

Although it is generally accepted that the One Health approach is essential for tackling antimicrobial resistance, the relative contribution of animals, food, the environment and the human population is still poorly understood. Nevertheless, it is beyond doubt that reduction of antimicrobial resistance in animal production systems contributes to reduction in the global spread of antimicrobial resistance.

During the 2023 AMR workshop in Amsterdam, different breakout sessions were organized, in which the impact of antimicrobial usage in animals on antimicrobial resistance in animals and humans was discussed as well as different options to reduce antimicrobial use in livestock farming. This included governmental measures, farm management, hygiene, animal health and welfare, antibiotic alternatives and artificial intelligence. This chapter provides an overview of the main outcomes of these break-out session combined with a review of the scientific literature on these subjects.

Keywords Resistance prevention · AMR interventions · AMR development AMR spreading · Livestock health care

Introduction

Antimicrobial resistance is generally recognized as a major public health issue. Globally more antimicrobials are used for livestock than for humans (Sucena Afonso et al. 2024). Fortunately, monitoring of resistance in those areas where

L. P. Carmo
Norwegian Veterinary Institute, Ås, Norway

Veterinary Public Health Institute, Liebefeld, Switzerland

Vetsuisse Faculty, University of Bern, Liebefeld, Switzerland
e-mail: luis.gomesdocarmo@unibe.ch

K. D. C. Stärk
Federal Food Safety and Veterinary Office, Liebefeld, Switzerland
e-mail: katharina.staerk@blv.admin.ch

B. ter Kuile
Swammerdam Institute of Life Sciences, University of Amsterdam, Amsterdam, The Netherlands
e-mail: b.h.terkuile@uva.nl

prudent veterinary use is enforced indicates that, the prevalence of resistance no longer increases and sometimes even starts to decrease (EFSA/ECDC 2024; Veldman et al. 2024). This development demonstrates that rules and regulations for the application of antibiotics are valuable tools to counter antimicrobial resistance. Of the total incidence of ESBL in human pathogens, about one quarter is originally selected in the agricultural sector (Mughini-Gras et al. 2019). It is not clear to what extent that attribution is also valid for other forms of antimicrobial resistance. In the case of ESBLs, model estimations suggest that without the continuous input from an undefined non-human sources, the prevalence in human pathogens would eventually go down to zero (Mughini-Gras et al. 2019). However, it is beyond dispute that some of the antimicrobial resistance encountered in human pathogens originates from livestock.

The most effective measures on reducing selection of antimicrobial resistance combine good farm management (including proper housing, hygiene and care for the animals) with an application methodology that prevents any unnecessary development and spreading of antimicrobial resistance. Simply said the best way to treat infections is using the highest dose that the animals can handle for the shortest time needed to clear the infection (Ter Kuile et al. 2016; Llewelyn et al. 2017). In that manner, the exposure of bacteria to non-lethal concentrations of antibiotics, the main driving factor for development and spreading of resistance, is prevented. The crucial matter is how to achieve that. Even the most detailed laws, such as the EU regulation 6/2019, contain lots of open standards and do not describe methods, but rather what must be achieved.

During the AMR workshop in Amsterdam in 2023, several subjects were discussed which are included in this review. Initially the possibilities to reduce usage of antibiotics are explored. In particular, food production sectors seem to offer room for improvement in the sense that adaptations at farms can reduce the need for treatment of infections. Subsequently the major challenges associated with hygiene and animal health and welfare are addressed. In the same framework, alternatives for antibiotics are considered. The extremely rapid developments in the area of artificial intelligence offer opportunities for almost all human activities, so it is logical to explore those for improving livestock production and particularly antimicrobial use practices as well. The assessment is rounded off with an analysis of the mechanisms behind the spread of antimicrobial resistance from animals to humans to focus on the most profitable avenues of action regarding improvement and innovation aiming at reducing the disease load caused by antimicrobial resistance.

Impact of Antimicrobial Usage in Animals on Antimicrobial Resistance in Humans

Factors Affecting the Relationship Between Antimicrobial Usage and Antimicrobial Resistance in Animals

The impact of antimicrobial usage in food producing animals on antimicrobial resistance in humans depends on several factors. Focusing on the animal sector, it is important to understand the relation between antimicrobial usage and antimicrobial resistance. Although the variation in biological mechanisms behind development of antimicrobial resistance is wide and not fully understood (Reygaert 2018), the association between antimicrobial usage and antimicrobial resistance has been shown in animal and human populations (Bell et al. 2014; Holmes et al. 2016; EFSA-ECDC 2024). Interventions reducing antimicrobial usage in animals are associated with decreased antimicrobial resistance in animals and humans (Tang et al. 2017). In the Netherlands, antimicrobial usage in animals was reduced substantially over the last decades. A combination of voluntary and compulsory measures implemented in the Dutch livestock sector in 2009/2010 (Speksnijder et al. 2015), resulted in a more than 77% reduction of sales of antimicrobials in 2022 (Heederik et al. 2023). Antimicrobial resistance is reported yearly for European countries (EFSA) and also on national level (e.g. MARAN in the Netherlands). The data show decreasing trends of antimicrobial resistance in indicator bacteria (commensals and pathogens) in most food producing animals over the last years (EFSA-ECDC 2024; Veldman et al. 2024). However, this does not hold for all pathogens, e.g. high levels of resistance for fluoroquinolones and tetracyclines were still found in *Campylobacter* isolates from humans and poultry, and most pig farms are still LA-MRSA positive (van Duijkeren et al. 2025) despite reduction in usage of these specific antibiotics (Veldman et al. 2023). Critical success factors for the development and dissemination of resistance, both in humans and animals, depend on the bacteria involved, the selective pressure imposed by the use of antimicrobials and the transferability of resistance genes. Therefore, limited and correct use of antimicrobials is an important measure to counteract the development of antimicrobial resistance. This includes prescribing antimicrobials based on a correct diagnosis of the causative agent and valid antimicrobial susceptibility testing. An appropriate choice of antimicrobials should be based on guidelines. In the Netherlands these veterinary clinical practice guidelines are developed by the Royal Dutch Veterinary Association (KNMvD), that can be used, on a voluntary basis, by veterinarians to decide on a evidence-based recommendations on the diagnostics and treatment options (Formularia—WVAB). These recommendations are based on several considerations: 1) clinical effectivity of the antimicrobials, 2) indications for use as mentioned in the SPC, 3) limiting negative side-effects for both human and animal, 4) classification of first, second, third choice antimicrobials, 5) the aim to optimize effectivity of antimicrobials, and 6) limiting development and transmission of resistant bacteria and resistance genes. The EMA has published a report (AMEG

2018—Categorisation of antibiotics (europa.eu)) and infographic (Categorisation of antibiotics for use in animals (europa.eu)) as a tool to support decision making by veterinarians on antimicrobial prescription. This advice includes categorization of antibiotics based on potential consequences for human health in terms of antimicrobial resistance, which has also resulted in a list of antimicrobials exclusively for use in humans (Schmerold et al. 2023).

Next to the mentioned factors and mechanism of the relation between antimicrobial usage and antimicrobial resistance there are the social and economic issues of a society in which these processes occur. Given the concern about the development of antimicrobial resistance in different animal sectors, there is an increasing awareness with regard to antimicrobial usage which has been a driving force for reduction in antimicrobial usage in the Netherlands. Other factors that may influence antimicrobial usage by a farmer can be external pressure resulting in certain behavior, responsibility, and economic factors (Coyne et al. 2014). In addition, other actors in the production chain such as suppliers and buyers influence antimicrobial usage at the farm level. For the veterinarians the relation with their client is another influencing factor in the decision to use antimicrobials in particular situations (Coyne et al. 2014; Wayop et al. 2024).

One of the measures implemented in the Dutch livestock sectors was the establishment of the independent Netherlands Veterinary Medicines Authority (SDa), responsible for analyzing, benchmarking and reporting yearly antimicrobial usage on farm and veterinarian level based on prescription data collected in national databases. Based on this, target levels for responsible use are set and high users and high prescribers can be identified. These are required to take additional efforts to reduce their use (Bos et al. 2015). Still, in some animal sectors, a substantial number of farms continuously fall within the category of 'high users'. The current Dutch policy on responsible antimicrobial use is to specifically focus on these high users (Heederik et al. 2023). As an example, intensive coaching of high user farms has shown to be effective in reducing antimicrobial usage (Caekebeke et al. 2021; McKernan et al. 2021).

The Relationship Between Antimicrobial Resistance in Animals and in Humans

The presence of antimicrobial resistance in food producing animals constitutes a threat for human health care. Several source attribution studies have investigated the contribution of animals to the presence of antimicrobial resistance in humans. Although most carriership in humans was attributed to human to human transmission, also food and contact with farm animals were defined as relevant sources with source attribution of 18.9% and 3.6%, respectively (Mughini-Gras et al. 2019). To which extend consumers are exposed to antimicrobial resistant bacteria in meat products depends on the type of meat and processing of the meat before consuming

(Evers et al. 2017). This also includes general kitchen/food hygiene. Also direct contact with (farm) animals has been considered as a risk factor for antimicrobial resistance carriage (Leverstein-van Hall et al. 2011), and contacts between wild animals and humans via a shared environment, like open water (Dorado-Garcia et al. 2018). Most of the studies mentioned above are based on the degree of similarity between the molecular characteristics of ESBL-producing *E. coli* from different sources. For most other resistance mechanisms and/or bacterial species fewer data are available. Another well-known example of a resistant bacterium that was thought to particularly spread from livestock to humans is the Livestock-Associated MRSA (LA-MRSA). However, a recent study describes an increase of a specific more pathogenic variant (PVL-positive-LA-MRSA) without a clear link to livestock (Witteveen et al. 2022). This indicates that LA-MRSA can thrive, develop and spread in humans without livestock as intermediate host. These results call for reconsideration of the name 'LA-MRSA'.

Several mechanisms cause the spread of antimicrobial resistance from animals to humans. Although the above mentioned source attribution studies focused on the genetic similarity between antimicrobial resistance in different sectors or sources, they do not distinguish between animal related isolates that temporarily colonise humans because of their shared environment or strains from animal origin that successfully and persistently colonise the human population. The transmission of antimicrobial resistance from animals to humans will have a higher potential risk for human health. In case animal isolates adapt to humans, new combinations of genes and plasmids might increase successful colonisation or even infect humans. Critical elements in these processes are the pathways and different levels of transmission of resistance, i.e. vertically via clonal spread, or horizontally via mobile elements such as plasmids or transposons, summarized as the spreading potential.

Improving Farm Management in the Context of AMR

Antimicrobial Stewardship at Farm Level

As there is a strong association between total AMU in (farm) animals and the development and potential spread of antimicrobial resistance (genes), it is of utmost importance to reduce total use of antimicrobials in farm animals and specifically the use those antimicrobial classes with the highest relevance to human health. Antimicrobials in farm animals should only be used when there is a significant benefit from using them which outweighs the risk of development and spread of antimicrobial resistance. Actually, Farm to Fork strategy set out that sale of antimicrobials for farmed animals and in aquaculture has to be reduced by 50% until 2023 (Commission 2025). Furthermore, emphasis must be placed on prudent and responsible antimicrobial use (Commission 2015), which can be achieved by implementing disease-specific guidelines. While some guidelines have already been developed, they need to be adopted and consistently applied at the national level due to countries specificities. A key concept here is Antimicrobial Stewardship which can be captured in the 5Rs framework of responsibility, reduction, replacement, refinement and review (Scott Weese et al. 2013). A strong pillar is reducing the risk of infectious diseases affecting production animals, as every bacterial infection prevented equals omission of an antimicrobial treatment as long as antimicrobials are not applied for prevention. The European Medicines Agency's (EMA) efforts to implement species-specific benchmarking AMU on farm level represent a crucial step forward in this area. Additionally, a significant advancement is the development of monitoring and surveillance systems for AMU in farm animals in low- and middle-income countries, especially non-EU countries.

Triad of Infections

The outcome of a (bacterial) infection is in its essence dependent on characteristics and the complex interplay between host, pathogen and environment whereby in the case of infections the pathogen continuously cycles around basic processes leading to association, multiplication, immune evasion, damage and transmission (Prescott 2022). An additional challenge in livestock systems is the fact that many disease complexes are multi-agent in nature whereby primary pathogens pave the way for more severe opportunistic infections (Prescott 2022). In order to prevent diseases, interventions are needed that break the cycle of infections, from early association (e.g. colonization, invasion) to transmission to another animal, targeting at least one of the classic elements of the historical triad being the host, environment or pathogen. Farmers, through preventive management approaches can, assisted by advice and interventions provided by their veterinarian, try to prevent infectious diseases as much as possible. These efforts not only enhance animal welfare and productivity but also contribute to broader public health goals by reducing the risk of antimicrobial resistance and ensuring the sustainability of animal agriculture.

Prevention of Infections

Classically, most interventions have focused on improving the host susceptibility to infection through the application of vaccinations, prevention of colonization and invasion by means of preventive antimicrobial treatment and measures to reduce transmission like improving biosecurity. There is a strong literature base for many farm-level (technical) interventions (e.g. improving internal and external biosecurity practices, improving feed quality, altering vaccination regimes, deviation from group treatments) that are either alone but mostly in combination able to reduce the need for antimicrobials (Speksnijder et al. 2015; Gozdzielewska et al. 2020; van Asseldonk et al. 2020; Pinto Jimenez et al. 2023). It should, however, be acknowledged that a one-size-fits-all-approach is never feasible. Each farm and veterinarian has its own context and unique mix of facilitators and barriers to reduce antimicrobial use. The implementation of preventive measures differs between countries. Most knowledge of effective management practices derives from high income countries and there is a worrisome lack of studies on effective antimicrobial stewardship interventions in middle- and lower income countries (Gozdzielewska et al. 2020; Pinto Jimenez et al. 2023). From experiences in countries like Denmark and the Netherlands who have known substantial reductions in veterinary AMU, it can be learned that although the 'low hanging fruit' has been harvested (i.e. the easy measures have mostly been applied), still there is room for improvement in implementing these existing measures on each farm by farmers and veterinarians. A way to achieve this could be through specific interventions focusing on implementation and using the social sciences to understand how human behavior can be altered. A few good examples in the veterinary field already exist (Morgans et al. 2021; Wayop et al. 2024). Moreover, tailored biosecurity plans that address the specific needs and challenges of each farm can lead to more sustainable and effective disease prevention. This can be achieved by using tools such as the Biocheck.UGent™ scoring tool (Gelaude et al. 2014; Tanquilut et al. 2020) which is easily applicable to farms regardless of the country's income level.

Challenges, Future Developments and Directions

Apart from improving implementation of current 'best practices' through addressing facilitators and barriers for change using multidisciplinary approaches, improvements can be made in technical interventions, and new approaches are possible with the use of sensor technology and artificial intelligence and rapid diagnostics.

Sensors applied in dairy farming are an example of a precision livestock farming tool measuring physiological, behavioral, and production indicators of individual animals to improve herd productivity, to assess general cattle health and monitor presence of disease. Hence, implementing this enhanced diagnostic tool can aid in the early detection and targeted treatment of infections, thereby reducing the blanket use of (broad-spectrum) antimicrobials.

Implementing strategies such as pharmacoeconomic analysis in veterinary medicine represents one of the promising approaches to promote more cost-effective and sustainable treatment options. By evaluating the economic benefits of alternative treatments, in comparison to conventional antibiotics, veterinarians and farmers can make more informed decisions that not only address the clinical efficacy of treatments but also optimize financial outcomes (Kovacevic et al. 2022a). Connection between AMU and AMR (Kovacevic et al. 2022b) reinforces the importance of evaluating and potentially adopting alternative non-antibiotic treatments (Tomanic et al. 2023), which may offer not only cost savings but also a reduction in the risk of AMR. Integrating pharmacoeconomic analyses with AMR data provides a comprehensive approach to improving mastitis management strategies, highlighting the need for continued research and implementation of effective, cost-saving and sustainable treatments in dairy farming, particularly in managing prevalent and costly diseases like bovine mastitis.

Many interventions aiming at supporting antimicrobial stewardship have focused on individual farms and veterinarians, rather than the impact of the wider and complex system of animal food production on antimicrobial use practices. Current food animal production systems are mostly built on economic profitability and efficiency with animal breeds specifically selected for maximum productivity. Increasingly we are confronted with possible negative tradeoffs in terms of animal welfare, environmental impacts (including climate) and also antimicrobial use, although it should be noticed that these effects are ambiguous and sometimes conflicting.

In poultry farming, broilers have for decades been selected for maximum growth and feed conversion and the current broiler production systems are extraordinarily efficient. However, the tradeoffs of this system in terms of animal welfare and antimicrobial use are increasingly recognized (Vissers et al. 2021). Future directions that require changes along the system rather than the individual farm could be the concept of slower growing broilers with lower stocking densities which significantly reduces the need for antimicrobial treatments and improves animal welfare, although it has its tradeoffs as well. This concept has been successfully adopted in the Netherlands under increasing public pressure where supermarkets nowadays only sell chicken meat from slower growing broilers with slightly lower stocking densities and farmers are paid a premium price (Vissers et al. 2021). In addition, the concept of on-farm hatching is promising as it improves animal welfare, gastrointestinal health and can lower antimicrobial use (Jerab et al. 2023). However, these changes go beyond the individual farm and require adaptations in the whole production chain.

Both piglets in the swine industry and non-breeding calves in the dairy industry are typically exposed to many stress factors early in life when they are still not immunocompetent. In pig farming, there is increasing evidence that early weaning (typically at 3–4 weeks) is associated with a higher antimicrobial use as longer suckling (5–7 weeks which comes closer to nature where weaning starts from 8 weeks onwards) provides more immunocompetent piglets with a higher viability, better intestinal health and better abilities to fight pathogens (Postma et al. 2016; Mallioris et al. 2024). Surplus dairy calves (or cross-bred calves) mostly are sent to the veal calf or beef industry at a very young age, often when they are only a couple of days or weeks old and in the middle of their 'immunity gap'. Examples of often encountered stressors that jeopardizes the immune system and exposes these young animals to a wide variety of pathogens are suboptimal colostrum provision on the dairy farm (leading to failure of passive transfer), transportation (including food and water deprivation) and comingling on the receiving farm (stress and massive exposure to pathogens) (Creutzinger et al. 2021; Webb et al. 2023). Future directions that will improve animal welfare and foster the resilience of these young calves and therewith reduce the need for antimicrobial treatments are amongst others to increase the minimum age of transport, try to eliminate assembly points and to reward dairy farmers for raising surplus calves of a higher quality (Webb et al. 2023). However, this also implicates a significant restructuring of existing production chains.

There is a strong need to rethink current livestock production systems comprehensively in light of animal welfare and health, environmental implications, antimicrobial use and resistance and economic profitability for farmers. This goes beyond the individual farm level and requires a holistic systems thinking approach with input from a wide variety of scientific disciplines. There often is a lack of knowledge among farm animal veterinarians regarding antimicrobial stewardship and its practical applications in managing antimicrobial resistance (Vidovic et al. 2022; Cobo-Angel et al. 2023) where key barriers were a lack of antimicrobial stewardship governance structures, client expectations and competition between practices, cost of microbiological testing, and lack of access to education, training and AMS resources (Hardefeldt et al. 2018). This gap highlights the need for more comprehensive and targeted educational initiatives. Hence, continuous education and training for farmers and veterinarians on antimicrobial stewardship principles are crucial for the sustainable use of antimicrobials in farm animals, ensuring both animal health and public safety.

Hygiene, Animal Health and Animal Welfare

What Are the Major Challenges Associated with Hygiene and Animal Health and Welfare?

As a global veterinary and public health threat, antimicrobial resistance has led national and international organisations to design and implement policies aimed at preserving the efficacy of antimicrobials. Many human and animal health policies focus on reducing the need for antibiotics through improved infection prevention and control (IPC), antibiotic stewardship, and research and development of new or alternative treatments and improved diagnostics. In animal health, reported challenges include a lack of alternatives to antibiotics, technical difficulties in infection control and prevention, diversity of farming systems, sustained behaviour change and compliance with health programmes, lack of clarity and misinformation on animal health and welfare standards, and in some cases increasing consumer pressure to stop using antibiotics altogether in livestock, poultry and aquaculture which would have serious negative consequences on animal health and welfare. Here we will focus on the following: animal health and welfare, infection prevention and control, hygiene and biosecurity measures as alternatives to antibiotic treatments.

Animal Health and Welfare

Biosecurity and hygiene are to reduce the spread of infection and infectious disease, thereby reducing the need for treatments in general and antibiotics in particular. The Food and Agriculture Organization of the United Nations (FAO) stated that improved health and welfare would make animals less prone to contract infectious diseases, thus minimising the need for antimicrobials (Magnusson et al. 2019). However, despite a number of reported benefits, it is challenging to quantify the impact of initiatives to improve animal health and welfare on the reduction of Antimicrobial Use (AMU) and AMR and there is a paucity of empirical evidence (Rodrigues da Costa and Diana 2022). Despite this, a recent study has indicated that a statistically significant lower AMU was observed where the level of welfare improved (Diana et al. 2020). In addition, (Rodrigues da Costa and Diana 2022) concluded that, in farm animals, better animal welfare often is associated with lower AMU, and that, generally, poor welfare is associated with higher AMU. It should be acknowledged however that this association often is complex and that withholding necessary treatments from sick animals can also jeopardise animal welfare.

Infection Prevention and Control

Infection prevention and control (IPC) is a scientific approach and practical solution designed to prevent harm caused by infection to patients and health workers in both animal and human healthcare settings. Therefore, maintaining high standards of hygiene and cleanliness in veterinary practice is vitally important to ensure the safety of patients, staff and clients by minimising the risk of acquiring infection whilst on the premises (Gerrard 2020). However, there is a paucity of studies available in the public domain that have investigated IPC in veterinary healthcare settings. Nevertheless, recent studies have started to employ the Theory of Interpersonal Behaviour as a comprehensive model for understanding the determinants of behaviour such as hand hygiene. In addition, recent studies have also explored the use of 3D animation to improve IPC in veterinary practices and hospitals (Macdonald et al. 2021). Maintaining high levels of biosecurity are also of paramount importance when considering IPC.

Alternatives to Antimicrobials

With the advent of the global antimicrobial resistance crisis, our arsenal of effective antimicrobials is rapidly diminishing (Betts et al. 2018). Consequently, alternatives to traditional antimicrobials are urgently needed. Although several novel strategies are under investigation, their efficacy and reliability for treating infections must be rigorously demonstrated. To date, none of these alternatives have shown efficacy comparable to curative antibiotic treatments. Emerging approaches can generally be categorised into two main groups: those that target specific bacterial pathogens and those that promote health by modulating the microbiome.

In this context, we explored available alternative strategies and their confirmed or anticipated efficacy to treat infections, as discussed during an expert workshop. Below, we describe these strategies.

A prominent approach gaining attention involves the administration of favourable bacteria or their derivatives, including probiotics (live microorganisms), prebiotics (non-viable substrates that serve as nutrients for beneficial bacteria), and postbiotics (compounds derived from non-living microorganisms), for prophylactic or therapeutic health improvement. Probiotics, for example, have shown success in lowering the faecal carriage of *Salmonella* and *Escherichia coli* in chickens (Nakamura et al. 2002; Nuotio et al. 2013). However, concerns remain regarding the efficacy and reproducibility of these interventions due to variations in the formulations and used experimental conditions (Allen 2017). Additionally, studies claiming efficacy against AMR-associated pathogens often suffer from methodological inconsistencies, variable readouts, and reliance on empirical clinical data (Suez et al. 2019). Similarly, for postbiotics, safety and potential adverse effects remain poorly characterised (Salminen et al. 2021). The lack of reliable information regarding mechanisms of action, appropriate dosing regimens, species- or age-specific responses and interactions between probiotics and other members of the microbiota, highlights the urgent need for further research to establish the efficacy and safety of these strategies.

An alternative approach to combating bacterial infections is the use of bacteriophages, viruses that specifically infect target bacteria by binding to unique bacterial receptors. This specificity requires detailed knowledge of the bacterial pathogen to select an appropriate phage, which complicates treatment compared to the broad-spectrum nature of conventional antimicrobials. Although in veterinary medicine phage therapy has been successful for reduction of *Salmonella* and *Campylobacter* shedding in poultry, and treatment of mastitis in cows (Ahmadi et al. 2016; Peh et al. 2023), there are also inconsistent results. Moreover, these studies are largely anecdotal with limited support from clinical trials (Verstappen et al. 2016; Loponte et al. 2021). Several challenges hinder the broader application of phage therapy. These include the potential development of phage resistance, the limited efficacy of phages in complex biological matrices, and interactions with the host immune system. Further research is needed to address these limitations and optimize phage-based therapeutic approaches. An alternative to phages is the use of phage-derived lysins, which are enzymes capable of specifically targeting bacterial pathogens. For example, lysins targeting *Staphylococcus aureus* have shown promise in treating skin infections. However, their potential effects on the microbiota and their overall efficacy in treating infections are not yet fully supported by current data (Fischetti 2018; Xu 2021). Currently there is still no specific legislation that regulates the use of phage therapy, although the European Medicines Agency recently published a guideline for phage therapy (EMA/CVMP/NTWP/32862/2022), more studies on safety and efficacy of phages are required.

Dietary interventions present another promising approach to reducing the reliance on antimicrobials. These interventions include fermented foods, fiber-rich diets, acidifiers, phytochemicals, and metals, which aim to modulate microbial ecosystems and activate immune cells on mucosal and cutaneous surfaces. Such strategies are designed to lower the risk of disease and enhance overall health (Allen 2017; Betts et al. 2018). By promoting a balanced microbial environment and reducing infection rates, dietary interventions can help decrease antimicrobial usage. This reduction, in turn, minimizes the selective pressure that drives the emergence and transmission of antibiotic resistance genes. However, despite their potential, further research is needed to elucidate the mechanisms through which dietary interventions contribute to health. Understanding these mechanisms will be critical for optimizing these strategies and integrating them effectively into veterinary and human healthcare.

While challenges persist, ongoing research, and collaborative efforts are crucial for integrating probiotics, phage therapy and dietary interventions into mainstream clinical practice.

The pragmatic use of vaccines to protect against infectious diseases also contributes to reducing the use of antimicrobials and thus AMR.

How to Measure the Impact of Interventions to Prevent AMR

The underlying complexity in the epidemiology of antimicrobial resistance hampers thorough and comprehensive evaluations of the impact of interventions. Such an exercise becomes even more difficult to execute when the goal is to assess the impact that interventions implemented at farm level might have on public health, i.e. the indirect impact in a sector that is separate from where the interventions were applied. The report JIACRA IV—2019–2021 (EFSA/ECDC 2024) investigated the evidence available for different combinations of bacteria and antimicrobials on the links between antimicrobial consumption and resistance. One of the conclusions was that further targeted studies were needed to establish these associations.

Nonetheless, in an environment of limited resources, it is important to adequately evaluate the effect of interventions in order to prioritise implementation of policies that lead to the desired results (outcomes). In the context relevant here, an example of an outcome could be the reduction of the occurrence of AMR genes in the public health sector that emerged in the animal food-production systems. The methodology to measure the impact of preventive interventions in the livestock sector can be grouped into four themes. These are described below in the context of the scientific literature.

Pathway to Impact

The epidemiology of antimicrobial resistance is complex, and the participants acknowledged the existence of numerous data and knowledge gaps. This is in line with the scientific literature (Pinto Ferreira 2017; McCubbin et al. 2021; Guenin et al. 2023). The gaps stated by the participants encompassed the need for enhanced antimicrobial use and resistance data at the farm level, improved resistance data concerning antimicrobial resistance in animal-derived food, a comprehensive understanding of the livestock industry's contribution to the overall resistome, and its consequential impact on human health.

While surveillance activities may address some identified information needs, a substantial portion necessitates hypothesis-driven studies to understand the driving factors for resistance. The need for targeted research, namely to better understand transmission pathways and to unveil causation structures, has also been stressed in the latest JIACRA IV—2019–2021 (EFSA/ECDC 2024). Participants concurred on the imperative to gain a deeper understanding of the source attribution of resistant pathogens in public health. The relevance of source attribution information for risk managers has been stressed by Pires and colleagues (2018). The same authors have also identified challenges for its application within the context of AMR. These included the definition of the hazard and the lack of evidence to inform dose-response relationships. Despite the absence of information about source attribution, participants emphasized that decision-makers and health managers should not succumb to "intervention paralysis": antimicrobial resistance and the potential risk posed by the livestock industry must be managed.

The use of a theory-of-change approach to specify the pathways to impact was proposed as a strategic method to inform policy in the presence of knowledge gaps. This approach would help identify the information needs and could inform the prioritisation and design of additional studies to fill the gaps. Guenin and coworkers (2023) conducted a scoping review with the goal to identify "existing successful interventions in livestock that aimed at changing AMU to understand "what works, how, for whom, and why". While Guenin et al. (2023) looked at the success of an intervention as the change in practice towards a reduced or more prudent use of antimicrobials, we advocate that a similar approach can be taken to investigate outcomes along the food-production chain and up to the public health outcomes.

Execution of Intervention Studies

Aligned with the imperative to bridge knowledge gaps, participants of the workshop suggested the implementation of intervention studies, both at the farm and population levels. The latter, particularly pertinent for gauging the impact of policies, holds significance in advancing evidence-based practices throughout various steps of the food chain.

The need for intervention studies is supported by the literature. It is one of the pillars of the One Health priority research agenda for AMR by the WHO (Jesudason 2023; WHO 2023). Jacobsen and colleagues (Jacobsen et al. 2023) conducted a scoping review on antimicrobial resistance interventions in the animal sector. For the authors, the lack of intervention research was particularly worrisome in low-and-middle income countries. Also, the need for economic evaluation was stressed as a relevant indicator to assess the feasibility of interventions. Tang and colleagues (Tang et al. 2017) reviewed the literature regarding the effect that restricting antimicrobial use in animals can have on AMR in animals and humans. The authors concluded that there is a low number of studies linking agricultural use to public health, which hampers a clear interpretation of the implications of such interventions.

Design Evaluation Plans for Interventions A Priori

Participants of the workshop highlighted the current lack of comprehensive evaluation strategies for interventions targeting antimicrobial resistance. Typically, evaluations are conducted retrospectively and can reveal important results. For example, an evaluation of the implementation of the 2013–2018 UK national AMR strategy provided relevant information for a refresh of the strategy for 2019–2024, namely by looking into the effectiveness of the interventions and relevant gaps in actions addressing AMR and AMU (Blake et al. 2022).

However, the participants' perception was that when evaluations are conducted, they are often not planned prospectively, which can result in a lack of availability of data that would be needed. There was a consensus on the critical need to establish *a priori* design evaluation plans to better assess the impact of measures and policies along the pathway of resistance emergence and transmission from animals to humans. Well-structured and -executed evaluations were deemed pivotal for adequately assessing the efficacy of measures and policies. Tang and coworkers (Tang et al. 2017) highlighted the need to also investigate potential unintended consequences of interventions targeting AMU restrictions in the animal sector. This concern holds true for other interventions focused on curbing AMR and it is of particular relevance when operating in a One Health context, as the implementation of a measure in a given sector might have repercussions in others.

The Importance of Social Sciences

Participants of the workshop widely advocated for the incorporation of social sciences into the discourse. Recognising that social sciences can illuminate human behavioural aspects influencing the selection and spread of resistant bacteria, participants stressed the importance of collaborating with scientists and practitioners in this field. Such trans-disciplinary collaboration was seen as essential for gaining a nuanced understanding of the applicability and effectiveness of measures and policies. The participants' plea is supported widely in the literature (Magouras et al. 2017; Frid-Nielsen et al. 2019; Lu et al. 2020). Specific research needs related to behavioural insights and change were also identified through an international expert panel (WHO 2023). It is also documented that social science aspects, such as the personality of a farmer, can have a direct impact on AMU and therefore AMR.

Innovative Approaches to Reduce AMU and AMR Using a Systemic Approach

How Can Artificial Intelligence Be Used to Improve Animal Health and Welfare?

Artificial intelligence (AI) and machine learning (ML) have the potential to revolutionise the animal health sector. There are opportunities for AI and ML to be applied in a number of animal health sectors to enhance health and welfare, including, improving the accuracy of diagnostics and clinical decision making (Beaudoin et al. 2016; Rai et al. 2022, 2024; Morisi et al. 2023; Poirier et al. 2023), R&D, for drug administration (e.g. improved dosatron accuracy), enhancing biosecurity and farm management practices based on seasonality and risk factors, alongside monitoring animal behaviour using remote and body sensors.

One area that is of particular interest is the role of AI and ML in tackling antimicrobial resistance, and its application in antimicrobial drug development, prediction of antimicrobial resistance, and antibiotic stewardship. With the reduction in sequencing price and acceleration of sequencing speed, it is now possible to accurately and directly link the genotype and phenotype of bacteria (Tang et al. 2022; Wang et al. 2022a, b). Here we focus on the use of AI and ML to predict antimicrobial resistance in bacteria and its application in improving diagnostics for AMR.

Use of Machine Learning and AI to Predict Antimicrobial Resistance

Misuse of antibiotics is a key driving force for the development of AMR. Antibiotic prescriptions should be based on Antibiotic Sensitivity Testing, AST, to ensure the appropriate antibiotic is used. However, obtaining test results takes days and in many cases rapid clinical intervention is required before the results are received.

With the recent advances in sequencing technologies, applying Artificial Intelligence (AI) and Machine Learning (ML) techniques to predict AMR have resulted in promising outcomes such as improved accuracy and better workflow. However, there are challenges with multi-drug AMR prediction and in cases where samples are missing labels (Tharmakulasingam et al. 2023a). Recent studies have focused on using ML for antimicrobial stewardship by utilising data (treatments, treatment response etc.), extracted from hospital electronic health records, which can be done in real-time, and a similar approach has been proposed for dairy farms (Tharmakulasingam et al. 2023b).

Recent studies have used machine learning (ML) for predicting antibiotic sensitivity testing, AST (Smith et al. 2017), and predicting minimum inhibitory concentrations, MIC (Nguyen et al. 2019; Pataki et al. 2020; Wang et al. 2022a, b). In the study conducted by Nguyen et al. the model predicted Minimum Inhibitory Concentrations (MICs) with an overall average accuracy of 95%. The model used in the studies, predicted MICs with no *a priori* information about the underlying gene content or resistance phenotypes of the strains analysed (Nguyen et al. 2019). The recent progress in Whole Genome Sequencing (WGS) technology (better quality, increased speed and reduced cost) in combination with the availability of robust AI and ML approaches, indicates that WGS of bacteria might become cheaper and faster than undertaking basic disc diffusion and MIC assays.

To date, retrospective methodology for model development, nonstandard data processing and scarcity of validation in a randomised controlled trial or real-world studies, limit the application of these models in clinical practice (Tang et al. 2022). In addition, expert supervision, and the need for transparency and accountability when using AI to guide clinical decision making, and treatment choices are further considerations regarding the use of AI in clinical settings (Liu et al. 2024).

References

Ahmadi M, Karimi Torshizi MA, Rahimi S, Dennehy JJ (2016) Prophylactic bacteriophage administration more effective than post-infection administration in reducing Salmonella enterica serovar Enteritidis shedding in quail. Front Microbiol 7:1253

Allen HK (2017) Alternatives to antibiotics: why and how. NAM Perspectives

Beaudoin M, Kabanza F, Nault V, Valiquette L (2016) Evaluation of a machine learning capability for a clinical decision support system to enhance antimicrobial stewardship programs. Artif Intell Med 68:29–36

Bell BG, Schellevis F, Stobberingh E, Goossens H, Pringle M (2014) A systematic review and meta-analysis of the effects of antibiotic consumption on antibiotic resistance. BMC Infect Dis 14:13

Betts JW, Hornsey M & La Ragione RM (2018) Novel antibacterials: alternatives to traditional antibiotics. Adv Microb Physiol 73: 123–169, Elsevier

Blake LJ, Häsler B, Bennani H, Mateus AL, Eastmure E, Mays N, Stärk KD (2022) The UK antimicrobial resistance strategy 2013–18: a qualitative study of international and domestic policy and action related to livestock and the food chain. Front Sustain Food Syst 6

Bos ME, Mevius DJ, Wagenaar JA, van Geijlswijk IM, Mouton JW, Heederik DJ, Netherlands Veterinary Medicines A (2015) Antimicrobial prescription patterns of veterinarians: introduction of a benchmarking approach. J Antimicrob Chemother 70:2423–2425

Caekebeke N, Ringenier M, Jonquiere FJ et al (2021) Coaching Belgian and Dutch broiler farmers aimed at antimicrobial stewardship and disease prevention. Antibiotics 10

Cobo-Angel C, Roche SM, LeBlanc SJ (2023) Understanding the role of veterinarians in antimicrobial stewardship on Canadian dairy farms: a mixed-methods study. PLoS One 18:e0289415
Commission E (2015) Guidelines for the prudent use of antimicrobials in veterinary medicine
Commission E (2025) Farm to fork strategy
Coyne LA, Pinchbeck GL, Williams NJ, Smith RF, Dawson S, Pearson RB, Latham SM (2014) Understanding antimicrobial use and prescribing behaviours by pig veterinary surgeons and farmers: a qualitative study. Vet Rec 175:593
Creutzinger K, Pempek J, Habing G, Proudfoot K, Locke S, Wilson D, Renaud D (2021) Perspectives on the management of surplus dairy calves in the United States and Canada. Front Vet Sci 8:661453
Diana A, Lorenzi V, Penasa M, Magni E, Alborali GL, Bertocchi L, De Marchi M (2020) Effect of welfare standards and biosecurity practices on antimicrobial use in beef cattle. Sci Rep 10:20939
Dorado-Garcia A, Smid JH, van Pelt W et al (2018) Molecular relatedness of ESBL/AmpC-producing Escherichia coli from humans, animals, food and the environment: a pooled analysis. J Antimicrob Chemother 73:339–347
EFSA/ECDC (2024) JIACRA 4 antimicrobial consumption and resistance in bacteria from humans and food-producing animals. EFSA J 172
EFSA-ECDC (2024) The European Union summary report on antimicrobial resistance in zoonotic and indicator bacteria from humans, animals and food in 2021–2022. EFSA J 195
Evers EG, Pielaat A, Smid JH, van Duijkeren E, Vennemann FB, Wijnands LM, Chardon JE (2017) Comparative exposure assessment of ESBL-producing Escherichia coli through meat consumption. PLoS One 12:e0169589
Fischetti VA (2018) Development of phage Lysins as novel therapeutics: a historical perspective. Viruses 10
Frid-Nielsen SS, Rubin O, Baekkeskov E (2019) The state of social science research on antimicrobial resistance. Soc Sci Med 242:112596
Gelaude P, Schlepers M, Verlinden M, Laanen M, Dewulf J (2014) Biocheck.UGent: a quantitative tool to measure biosecurity at broiler farms and the relationship with technical performances and antimicrobial use. Poult Sci 93:2740–2751
Gerrard E (2020) Infection control and hygiene: a guide to best practice. Vet Nurs J 35:38–41
Gozdzielewska L, King C, Flowers P, Mellor D, Dunlop P, Price L (2020) Scoping review of approaches for improving antimicrobial stewardship in livestock farmers and veterinarians. Prev Vet Med 180:105025
Guenin MJ, Studnitz M, Molia S (2023) Interventions to change antimicrobial use in livestock: a scoping review and an impact pathway analysis of what works, how, for whom and why. Prev Vet Med 220:106025
Hardefeldt LY, Gilkerson JR, Billman-Jacobe H, Stevenson MA, Thursky K, Bailey KE, Browning GF (2018) Barriers to and enablers of implementing antimicrobial stewardship programs in veterinary practices. J Vet Intern Med 32:1092–1099
Heederik DJJ, Bonten MJM, Geijlswijk IMv, Dijk AJvH-v, Mughini-Gras L, Sanders P (2023) Het gebruik van antibiotica bij landbouwhuisdieren in 2023
Holmes AH, Moore LS, Sundsfjord A, Steinbakk M, Regmi S, Karkey A, Guerin PJ, Piddock LJ (2016) Understanding the mechanisms and drivers of antimicrobial resistance. Lancet 387:176–187
Jacobsen A, Ogden J, Ekiri AB (2023) Antimicrobial resistance interventions in the animal sector: scoping review. Front Antibiot 2:1233698
Jerab JG, Chantziaras I, Van Limbergen T, Van Erum J, Boel F, Hoeven E, Dewulf J (2023) Antimicrobial use in on-farm hatching systems vs. traditional hatching systems: a case study. Animals (Basel) 13
Jesudason T (2023) A one health priority research agenda for AMR. Lancet Microbe 4:e769

Kovacevic Z, Mihajlovic J, Mugosa S, Horvat O, Tomanic D, Kladar N, Samardzija M (2022a) Pharmacoeconomic analysis of the different therapeutic approaches in control of bovine mastitis: phytotherapy and antimicrobial treatment. Antibiotics 12

Kovacevic Z, Samardzija M, Horvat O, Tomanic D, Radinovic M, Bijelic K, Vukomanovic AG, Kladar N (2022b) Is there a relationship between antimicrobial use and antibiotic resistance of the most common mastitis pathogens in dairy cows? Antibiotics 12

Leverstein-van Hall MA, Dierikx CM, Cohen Stuart J et al (2011) Dutch patients, retail chicken meat and poultry share the same ESBL genes, plasmids and strains. Clin Microbiol Infect 17:873–880

Liu GY, Yu D, Fan MM, Zhang X, Jin ZY, Tang C, Liu XF (2024) Antimicrobial resistance crisis: could artificial intelligence be the solution? Mil Med Res 11:7

Llewelyn MJ, Fitzpatrick JM, Darwin E, SarahTonkin C, Gorton C, Paul J, Peto TEA, Yardley L, Hopkins S, Walker AS (2017) The antibiotic course has had its day. BMJ 358:j3418

Loponte R, Pagnini U, Iovane G, Pisanelli G (2021) Phage therapy in veterinary medicine. Antibiotics 10

Lu J, Sheldenkar A, Lwin MO (2020) A decade of antimicrobial resistance research in social science fields: a scientometric review. Antimicrob Resist Infect Control 9:178

Macdonald A, Chambers M, La Ragione R, Wyles K, Poyade M, Wales A, Klepacz N, Kupfer N, Watson F, Noble S (2021) Addressing infection risk in veterinary practice through the innovative application of interactive 3D animation methods. Des J 24:51–72

Magnusson U, Sternberg S, Eklund G, Rozstalnyy A (2019) Prudent and efficient use of antimicrobials in pigs and poultry, vol 23. FAO, Rome

Magouras I, Carmo LP, Stark KDC, Schupbach-Regula G (2017) Antimicrobial usage and -resistance in livestock: where should we focus? Front Vet Sci 4:148

Mallioris P, Luiken REC, Tobias T, Vonk J, Wagenaar JA, Stegeman A, Mughini-Gras L (2024) Risk factors for antimicrobial use in Dutch pig farms: a cross-sectional study. Res Vet Sci 174:105307

McCubbin KD, Anholt RM, de Jong E et al (2021) Knowledge gaps in the understanding of antimicrobial resistance in Canada. Front Public Health 9:726484

McKernan C, Benson T, Farrell S, Dean M (2021) Antimicrobial use in agriculture: critical review of the factors influencing behaviour. JAC Antimicrob Resist 3:dlab178

Morgans LC, Bolt S, Bruno-McClung E, van Dijk L, Escobar MP, Buller HJ, Main DCJ, Reyher KK (2021) A participatory, farmer-led approach to changing practices around antimicrobial use on UK farms. J Dairy Sci 104:2212–2230

Morisi A, Rai T, Bacon NJ, Thomas SA, Bober M, Wells K, Dark MJ, Aboellail T, Bacci B, La Ragione RM (2023) Detection of necrosis in digitised whole-slide images for better grading of canine soft-tissue sarcomas using machine-learning. Vet Sci 10

Mughini-Gras L, Dorado-Garcia A, van Duijkeren E et al (2019) Attributable sources of community-acquired carriage of Escherichia coli containing beta-lactam antibiotic resistance genes: a population-based modelling study. Lancet Planet Health 3:e357–e369

Nakamura A, Ota Y, Mizukami A, Ito T, Ngwai YB, Adachi Y (2002) Evaluation of aviguard, a commercial competitive exclusion product for efficacy and after-effect on the antibody response of chicks to salmonella. Poult Sci 81:1653–1660

Nguyen M, Long SW, McDermott PF, Olsen RJ, Olson R, Stevens RL, Tyson GH, Zhao S, Davis JJ (2019) Using machine learning to predict antimicrobial MICs and associated genomic features for nontyphoidal salmonella. J Clin Microbiol 57

Nuotio L, Schneitz C, Nilsson O (2013) Effect of competitive exclusion in reducing the occurrence of Escherichia coli producing extended-spectrum beta-lactamases in the ceca of broiler chicks. Poult Sci 92:250–254

Pataki BA, Matamoros S, van der Putten BCL et al (2020) Understanding and predicting ciprofloxacin minimum inhibitory concentration in Escherichia coli with machine learning. Sci Rep 10:15026

Peh E, Szott V, Reichelt B, Friese A, Rosler U, Plotz M, Kittler S (2023) Bacteriophage cocktail application for campylobacter mitigation – from in vitro to in vivo. BMC Microbiol 23:209

Pinto Ferreira J (2017) Why antibiotic use data in animals needs to be collected and how this can be facilitated. Front Vet Sci 4:213

Pinto Jimenez CE, Keestra S, Tandon P, Cumming O, Pickering AJ, Moodley A, Chandler CIR (2023) Biosecurity and water, sanitation, and hygiene (WASH) interventions in animal agricultural settings for reducing infection burden, antibiotic use, and antibiotic resistance: a one health systematic review. Lancet Planet Health 7:e418–e434

Pires SM, Duarte AS, Hald T (2018) Source attribution and risk assessment of antimicrobial resistance. Microbiol Spectr 6

Poirier AC, Riano Moreno RD, Takaindisa L et al (2023) VIDIIA hunter diagnostic platform: a low-cost, smartphone connected, artificial intelligence-assisted COVID-19 rapid diagnostics approved for medical use in the UK. Front Mol Biosci 10:1144001

Postma M, Backhans A, Collineau L et al (2016) Evaluation of the relationship between the biosecurity status, production parameters, herd characteristics and antimicrobial usage in farrow-to-finish pig production in four EU countries. Porcine Health Manag 2:9

Prescott JF (2022) Themes in bacterial pathogenesis. In: Pathogenesis of bacterial infections in animals, pp 1–14

Rai T, Morisi A, Bacci B, Bacon NJ, Dark MJ, Aboellail T, Thomas SA, Bober M, La Ragione R, Wells K (2022) Deep learning for necrosis detection using canine perivascular wall tumour whole slide images. Sci Rep 12:10634

Rai T, Morisi A, Bacci B, Bacon NJ, Dark MJ, Aboellail T, Thomas SA, La Ragione RM, Wells K (2024) Keeping pathologists in the loop and an adaptive F1-score threshold method for mitosis detection in canine perivascular wall tumours. Cancers (Basel) 16

Reygaert WC (2018) An overview of the antimicrobial resistance mechanisms of bacteria. AIMS Microbiol 4:482–501

Rodrigues da Costa M, Diana A (2022) A systematic review on the link between animal welfare and antimicrobial use in captive animals. Animals (Basel) 12

Salminen S, Collado MC, Endo A et al (2021) The International Scientific Association of Probiotics and Prebiotics (ISAPP) consensus statement on the definition and scope of postbiotics. Nat Rev Gastroenterol Hepatol 18:649–667

Schmerold I, van Geijlswijk I, Gehring R (2023) European regulations on the use of antibiotics in veterinary medicine. Eur J Pharm Sci 189:106473

Scott Weese J, Page SW, Prescott JF (2013) Antimicrobial stewardship in animals. In: Antimicrobial therapy in veterinary medicine. Wiley, pp 117–132

Smith KP, Richmond DL, Brennan-Krohn T, Elliott HL, Kirby JE (2017) Development of MAST: a microscopy-based antimicrobial susceptibility testing platform. SLAS Technol 22:662–674

Speksnijder DC, Mevius DJ, Bruschke CJ, Wagenaar JA (2015) Reduction of veterinary antimicrobial use in The Netherlands. The Dutch success model. Zoonoses Public Health 62(Suppl 1):79–87

Sucena Afonso J, El Tholth M, McIntyre KM, Carmo LP, Coyne L, Manriquez D, Raboisson D, Lhermie G, Rushton J (2024) Strategies to reduce antimicrobials in livestock and aquaculture, and their impact under field conditions: a structured scoping literature review. J Antimicrob Chemother 79:11–26

Suez J, Zmora N, Segal E, Elinav E (2019) The pros, cons, and many unknowns of probiotics. Nat Med 25:716–729

Tang KL, Caffrey NP, Nobrega DB et al (2017) Restricting the use of antibiotics in food-producing animals and its associations with antibiotic resistance in food-producing animals and human beings: a systematic review and meta-analysis. Lancet Planet Health 1:e316–e327

Tang R, Luo R, Tang S, Song H, Chen X (2022) Machine learning in predicting antimicrobial resistance: a systematic review and meta-analysis. Int J Antimicrob Agents 60:106684

Tanquilut NC, Espaldon MVO, Eslava DF, Ancog RC, Medina CDR, Paraso MGV, Domingo RD, Dewulf J (2020) Quantitative assessment of biosecurity in broiler farms using Biocheck.UGent in Central Luzon, Philippines. Poult Sci 99:3047–3059
Ter Kuile BH, Kraupner N, Brul S (2016) The risk of low concentrations of antibiotics in agriculture for resistance in human health care. FEMS Microbiol Lett 363
Tharmakulasingam M, Gardner B, La Ragione R, Fernando A (2023a) Rectified classifier chains for prediction of antibiotic resistance from multi-labelled data with missing labels. IEEE/ACM Trans Comput Biol Bioinform 20:625–636
Tharmakulasingam M, Wang W, Kerby M, La Ragione R, Fernando A (2023b) TransAMR: an interpretable transformer model for accurate prediction of antimicrobial resistance using antibiotic administration data, vol 11. IEEE Access
Tomanic D, Kladar N, Radinovic M, Stancic I, Erdeljan M, Stanojevic J, Galic I, Bijelic K, Kovacevic Z (2023) Intramammary ethno-Veterinary formulation in bovine mastitis treatment for optimization of antibiotic use. Pathogens 12
van Asseldonk M, de Lauwere C, Bonestroo J, Bondt N, Bergevoet R (2020) Antibiotics use versus profitability on sow farms in The Netherlands. Prev Vet Med 178:104981
van Duijkeren E, Brouwer MSM, Wullings B et al (2025) Methicillin-resistant Staphylococcus aureus GG0398 on livestock farms and meat in The Netherlands. J Glob Antimicrob Resist 43:79–85
Veldman KT, Wit B, Franz E, Heederik DJJ (2023) Monitoring of antimicrobial resistance and antibiotic usage in animals in The Netherlands in 2022. Wageningen Bioveterinary Research (WBVR), Lelystad, p 76
Veldman KT, Wit B, Franz E, Heederik DJJ (2024) Maran 2024 monitoring of antimicrobial resistance and antibiotic usage in animals in The Netherlands in 2023. Wageningen Bioveterinary Research, Wageningen, p 77
Verstappen KM, Tulinski P, Duim B, Fluit AC, Carney J, van Nes A, Wagenaar JA (2016) The effectiveness of bacteriophages against methicillin-resistant Staphylococcus aureus ST398 nasal colonization in pigs. PLoS One 11:e0160242
Vidovic J, Stojanovic D, Cagnardi P, Kladar N, Horvat O, Cirkovic I, Bijelic K, Stojanac N, Kovacevic Z (2022) Farm animal veterinarians' knowledge and attitudes toward antimicrobial resistance and antimicrobial use in the Republic of Serbia. Antibiotics 11
Vissers LS, Saatkamp HW, Lansink AGO (2021) Analysis of synergies and trade-offs between animal welfare, ammonia emission, particulate matter emission and antibiotic use in Dutch broiler production systems. Agric Syst 189:103070
Wang S, Zhao C, Yin Y, Chen F, Chen H, Wang H (2022a) A practical approach for predicting antimicrobial phenotype resistance in Staphylococcus aureus through machine learning analysis of genome data. Front Microbiol 13:841289
Wang Y, Han Y, Li L, Liu J, Yan X (2022b) Distribution, sources, and potential risks of antibiotic resistance genes in wastewater treatment plant: a review. Environ Pollut 310:119870
Wayop IYA, de Vet E, Leerlooijer JN, Wagenaar JA, Speksnijder DC (2024) Using implementation mapping to develop an intervention program to support veterinarians' adherence to the guideline on Streptococcus suis clinical practice in weaned pigs. PLoS One 19:e0299905
Webb LE, Verwer C, Bokkers EA (2023) The future of surplus dairy calves – an animal welfare perspective. Front Anim Sci 4
WHO (2023) A one health priority research agenda for antimicrobial resistance.
Witteveen S, Hendrickx APA, de Haan A et al (2022) Genetic characteristics of methicillin-resistant Staphylococcus argenteus isolates collected in the Dutch national MRSA surveillance from 2008 to 2021. Microbiol Spectr 10:e0103522
Xu Y (2021) Phage and phage lysins: new era of bio-preservatives and food safety agents. J Food Sci 86:3349–3373

[illegible]

Chapter 3
Consequences of Antimicrobial Residuals in the Environment

Amy Pruden, Rebekah Riddle, Katherine Scott, and Ivan Odur

Abstract Antimicrobial residuals are not completely metabolized when administered to humans and animals and are excreted in urine and feces. Human waste is typically routed to a wastewater treatment plant, or on-site waste management systems for small communities, neither of which effectively remove antibiotics. Livestock wastes are subject to a variety of waste treatment processes, including composting, lagoons, and anaerobic digestion, which also marginally remove antimicrobials. Antibiotics and other antimicrobials thus can make their way into aquatic and soil environments as a result of use in human and veterinary medicine. Along the way from ingestion, to excretion, to waste collection, treatment, and discharge, antimicrobials can exert selection pressure and favor the evolution of antibiotic resistance genes (ARGs), horizontal gene transfer of ARGs among bacteria, and differential survival of bacteria carrying ARGs. Here we examine the potential consequences of antimicrobial residuals along these pathways, means to measure these consequences, and mitigate them. Animal and human waste treatment processes are important barriers to the spread of antimicrobial resistance to the environment and there are opportunities to continue to intentionally improve these processes intentionally for this purpose. At the same time, judicious use of antimicrobials is an essential means of limiting their release to the environment in the first place, but regulations and their enforcement varies internationally. Aquaculture systems are an example where there is particular vulnerability, given that antimicrobials are added directly to the water and also the international scale of trade in this industry. Direct release of antibiotics by pharmaceutical manufacturing industries is also a concern.

A. Pruden (✉) · K. Scott
Department of Civil & Environmental Engineering, Virginia Tech, Blacksburg, VA, USA
e-mail: apruden@vt.edu; kds145@vt.edu

R. Riddle
School of Public and International Affairs, Virginia Tech, Blacksburg, VA, USA
e-mail: becki417@vt.edu

I. Odur
Genetics, Bioinformatics, and Computational Biology, Virginia Tech, Blacksburg, VA, USA
e-mail: oivan@vt.edu

B. ter Kuile (ed.), *Antimicrobial Resistance and Antibiotics Usage in Livestock*,
https://doi.org/10.1007/978-3-032-04598-0_3

Efforts to determine the minimal selective concentrations (MSCs) and predicted no effect levels (PNECs) of antimicrobials and their mixtures in environmental settings can help to inform effective regulations for the judicious use of antibiotics and associated discharge of waste streams containing antimicrobials.

Keywords Antimicrobial resistance · Environment · Waste-water-treatment · Aquaculture · Minimal selective concentration

Objective of the White Paper

Antibiotics revolutionized the ability to prevent and treat deadly bacterial infections and embody one of the greatest scientific discoveries of the twentieth century. Together with vaccination and improved sanitation to prevent the spread of disease, human and animal health standards have greatly advanced. Antibiotics used in practice today are largely derived from natural sources, including secondary metabolites produced by microorganisms, along with chemically synthesized or partially synthesized compounds with similar properties (Demain and Sanchez 2009). Over the last century, antibiotics began to be mass produced and used routinely in human and veterinary medicine. This has resulted in human and animal gut microbes being routinely exposed to orders of magnitude higher concentrations of antibiotics than they had seen throughout prior evolutionary history. Likewise, excreted antibiotic parent compounds and metabolites will inevitably wind up in affected soil and aquatic environments. In AMR Session 1 of the "Conference on Optimal Practices to Protect Human Health Care from Antimicrobial Resistance Selected in the Veterinary Domain" held in Amsterdam October 2023, a discussion was convened to consider the potential negative consequences of antibiotics and other antimicrobials reaching the environment. Other antimicrobials included antifungals, antiparasitics, heavy metals, and other substances that generally act to kill or inhibit microbes, including bacteria and beyond. The **objective** of this white paper is to summarize the workshop discussion, in the context of relevant scientific literature, in order to highlight key unknowns and research needs.

The "impacts" of antimicrobials and their residues in the environment are somewhat distinct from the concern of traditional organic pollutants. There is scant evidence that antibiotics or antimicrobials, at typical environmental concentrations, cause any harm to ecosystems or their core functions (Huijbers et al. 2019). Rather, the concern is that clinical and veterinary use of antibiotics exerts selective pressure on corresponding gut microbiomes, resulting in differential survival and proliferation of antibiotic resistant bacteria (ARB) carrying antibiotic resistance genes (ARGs) (Aminov 2009). Further, ARGs can be shared amongst bacteria via horizontal gene transfer (HGT), particularly when carried on mobile genetic elements (MGE) such as integrons, plasmids, and prophages (Vikesland et al. 2019). Because of this, ARGs themselves can be considered to be environmental contaminants (Pruden et al. 2006). Lingering questions include exactly which antibiotics and what concentrations should be of concern for exerting selective pressure or inducing HGT when they are present in environments such as water and soil? Answers to such questions are critical to inform risk assessment and to support corresponding regulatory frameworks for discharge.

Here we first consider how antibiotics and other antimicrobials make their way into the environment, what impacts might be anticipated, and how this information might inform corresponding regulation and best practices aimed at mitigating the spread of antimicrobial resistance.

Pathways by Which Antibiotics and Other Antimicrobials Reach the Environment

Annually, several thousand tons of antimicrobials and their byproducts are estimated to be introduced into the environment. Antimicrobials may be released as a by-product of pharmaceutical manufacturing, wastestreams resulting from industrial use, excretion by humans, companion animals and livestock, direct application to crops, and disposal to landfills or other dumping sites. These sources can broadly be classified as point and non-point sources.

Point Sources and Their Treatment

Point sources largely include wastewater treatment plants (WWTPs) and industrial wastestreams. Landfills containing prescriptions that have been disposed of, and other sources are sometimes a point source, e.g., when the leachate is collected and routed to the WWTP for further treatment. For point sources, there is typically an opportunity to physically remove or chemically break down the active pharmaceutical ingredients (APIs) prior to discharge. However, treatment plants are often not intentionally designed for this purpose. Biological treatment is a highly effective means of removing organic pollutants from municipal wastewater and other wastestreams, but there are concerns regarding unanticipated negative consequences of involved in these processes being exposed to antimicrobials. The primary concern is that antimicrobials in the wastewater could exert selective pressure, resulting in selection and enrichment of resistant bacteria in the treated effluent. Fortunately, numerous surveys of WWTPs have demonstrated that in the vast majority of circumstances, antibiotic resistant bacteria (ARB) are largely reduced by conventional activated sludge wastewater treatment (Garner et al. 2024). However, there are some indications that specific ARB and antibiotic resistance genes (ARGs) are more sensitive to such selective pressure and thus should be more closely examined in future studies (Brown et al. 2024). Such concerns are amplified in pharmaceutical manufacturing and other industrial wastes, where the concentrations of APIs can occur in mixtures and at concentrations substantially higher than clinical breakpoints. Therefore, physical/chemical treatment, and not biological treatment, has been recommended for the treatment of pharmaceutical and industrial wastestreams (UNEP 2023). The ideal treatment will depend on the nature of the antibiotic/antimicrobial, including its stability, capacity to be oxidized or reduced, and capacity to be sorbed to media.

Point sources ultimately result in the discharge of antimicrobial residues that escape treatment into various aquatic environments, encompassing streams, rivers and lakes. Furthermore, during the reclamation of water for irrigation, these compounds can infiltrate soil and groundwater, potentially accumulating within soils, being absorbed by crops, or seeping into groundwater. In theory, point-sources are more readily controlled than non-point-sources.

Non-point Sources and the Mitigation

Non-point sources primarily encompass agricultural uses of antibiotics. Usage of antimicrobials in some fashion is largely viewed as essential to the contemporary agricultural sectors. An estimated 5393 tons of antibiotics were utilized in veterinary antimicrobials production in the European Union in 2004 (Kools et al. 2008). Globally, use in food animals is expected to increase by 8% by 2030 based on the current trends in use since 2020 (Mulchandani et al. 2023). Antibiotics are used to treat and prevent infectious disease in livestock and can be administered orally or via injection. Historically, antibiotics were used subtherapeutically to promote weight gain (Gelband et al. 2015), but this practice is falling out of favor, having been banned in the EU in 2006 and in the USA in 2017. Regardless of the purpose of use, some form of the parent API or metabolite will be excreted in the urine and feces of the livestock. Even though best practice administration of antimicrobials in the animal husbandry sector, about 40–90% of the antibiotics given to animals are excreted in the form of parent compounds, active metabolites, or conjugates (Jadeja and Worrich 2022; Lamshöft et al. 2007; Van Epps and Blaney 2016).

Livestock gut microbes are more likely to be enriched in ARB during antibiotic treatment and will be excreted along with the antimicrobial residues. This results in a challenge of manure management to reduce these residuals, but there are no specific guidelines specifically for reducing antimicrobial residues in manure. However, numerous studies have shown that antibiotics can be degraded or transformed during common manure management strategies, including stockpiling, composting (Chen et al. 2018), digestion (Wallace et al. 2018), or retention in lagoons (McKinney et al. 2010). Ultimately, non-point sources of antibiotics reach soil through application of treated or untreated manure. Antibiotics, ARB, and ARGs present in fertilizing or irrigation efforts, such as those in livestock manure, reclaimed water, and sewage can introduce antimicrobial residuals in the environment. (Hong et al. 2013). These can then be spread on crops as a form of fertilization or can leech into waterways through non-point source pollution from these farms (Hemamalini et al.

2022). Correspondingly, neighboring water bodies are impacted by runoff, during storm events.

Aquaculture represents a special case of an agricultural non-point source of antibiotics to the environment, where antibiotics are directly added to the water, which typically has connectivity with a natural water body. Biosolids, i.e., WWTP residuals, are also often land-applied in the same manner as manure, but will contain more human relevant antibiotics, ARB, and ARGs (Mays et al. 2021). Some antibiotics are also directly sprayed on crops. Antimicrobials in such scenarios disseminate through various pathways, including direct application on farms and aquacultures, improper disposal of containers and unused drugs, and through livestock feed. The excessive use of veterinary antimicrobials in livestock rearing significantly contributes to terrestrial antimicrobial residue pollution. Unlined landfills and dump sites additionally represent a non-point source of antibiotics not necessarily associated with agriculture.

Measuring the Environmental Impact of Antimicrobial Residuals

Analytical capabilities for detecting antibiotics in soil, water, wastewater, manure and other environmental samples came online in the late 1990s to early 2000s, largely due to advances in liquid chromatography and mass spectrometry (Aga et al. 2016). Such analysis is fundamentally challenging first due to difficulties separating and concentrating trace concentrations of very specific compounds. One approach to achieving this is through solid phase extraction (SPE), but inevitably it is not possible to achieve 100% efficient extraction, and efficiencies must be determined for each compound using positive controls. Also, it is difficult to identify and develop methods that are compatible with quantifying multiple antibiotics, and usually only a few can be quantified with a given method. More recently, non-targeted analysis is providing a means to screen hundreds of different pharmaceuticals of interest in a given sample, but the trade-off is lack of precise quantification (Manz et al. 2023).

Various studies have surveyed typical concentrations of a wide range of antibiotics used in human and animal populations in a wide array of environmental samples (Chow et al. 2021; Wilkinson et al. 2022). Generally, it is rare to encounter concentrations that are greater than those used in clinical applications to treat infections. A widely cited exception to this case was the pollution of a river in India with untreated pharmaceutical manufacturing waste, leading to concentrations of mixtures of antibiotics orders of magnitude above clinical break points (Larsson 2014). Correspondingly, it was not surprising to find DNA sequence evidence of MGE-associated ARGs in the river encoding resistance to last resort antibiotics of critical importance to human medicine (Kristiansson et al. 2011). Still, there are also concerns that sub-inhibitory levels of antibiotics could also exert selective pressure and stimulate mobility of ARGs (Chow et al. 2021).

Beyond measuring antibiotic compounds directly, being able to measure their impacts in the environment would provide direct guidance towards identifying discharge limits that limit risk of contributing to the evolution, selection, HGT, or persistence of antimicrobial resistance in the environment. Bioassays are one approach to demonstrating bioavailability of antibiotics (Aga et al. 2016). Since the advent of next generation DNA sequencing in the early 2010s, metagenomic sequencing is now providing a proxy for detecting changes in microbiomes and ARG profiles in response to antibiotics (Davis et al. 2023). Culture-based techniques, such as the World Health Organization's TriCycle protocol for extended-spectrum beta lactamase-producing *Escherichia coli* (WHO 2021), are useful for zeroing in on a viable clinical target of interest. However, it is difficult to relate outputs from low-throughput techniques to the complex array of environmental variables that could contribute to their occurrence. Otherwise, the general approach is to assume likely effects on environmental bacteria based on what is known about minimum inhibitory concentrations (MICs) for clinical bacteria from in vitro studies and selecting lowest concentrations with an observed effect, with a safety factor, to model predicted no effect concentrations (PNECs) (Bengtsson-Palme and Larsson 2016). However, given the complexity of microbial communities in the environments, it is not clear whether such a simplified approach is sufficient. The true no effect concentration can also change with time, with the passage of generations, for a given microbial community (Murray et al. 2018).

Various studies have documented effects of antibiotics on soil bacterial communities. Soils are the biggest reservoir of microbial biodiversity, but is also a large natural reservoir of ARGs. Multidrug-resistant soil bacteria contain ARGs to the main classes of medically important antibiotics found in human health, such as aminoglycosides, amphenicols, beta-lactams, sulfonamides, and tetracycline (Forsberg et al. 2012; Malagón-Rojas et al. 2020). Soils can transmit AMR to living organisms through a variety of pathways, including direct transmission, transmission via crops or livestock, and drinking water transmission (Jadeja and Worrich 2022). Thus, the main concern with impact to soil is whether antimicrobial and other additions increase the possibility of evolution and emergence of ARGs, and transmission of clinically-relevant ARGs into human pathogens.

The impact of antibiotic residues on the native microbial community's abundance and composition varies based on several factors including the type and quantity of antibiotic residues and the diversity of environmental microbes present (Grenni et al. 2018). For instance, investigations into the effects of tylosin and sulfadiazine have shown both short-term disturbance and enduring alterations in soil microbial community compositions, persisting even after antibiotic concentrations diminish. Thiele-Bruhn (2005) explored dose-dependent effects of sulfapyridine and oxytetracycline on microorganisms in various topsoils, revealing inhibitory doses at concentrations ranging from 0.003 to 7.35 $\mu g\ g^{-1}$ of total antibiotics. Moreover, antibiotics have been found to diminish soil bacterial populations and alter the fungal to bacterial ratio in a dose-dependent manner.

Similarly, antibiotic residues in aquatic environments, such as tetracycline at concentrations as low as 10 $\mu g\ L^{-1}$, can significantly impact the growth of

Synechocystis and *Lemna*. These residues not only alter the structure and abundance of soil microbial communities, but also affect their ability to degrade contaminants and fulfill ecological functions, like methanogenesis, nitrogen transformation, and sulfate reduction in both soil and aquatic ecosystems. For instance, the application of sulfadiazine-amended manure in soil has been observed to hinder nitrogen turnover processes and reduce microbial activity. In aquatic environments, oxytetracycline was found to inhibit nitrification even at low concentrations (12.5 mg L^{-1}), while sulfamethoxazole and ofloxacin inhibited methanogenesis in anaerobic digestion processes.

Potential for Human Exposure to Antibiotics via Environmental Sources and Implications

Reports indicate a direct correlation between human health and the environment, encompassing their living conditions and its various components, such as plants, animals, microorganisms, and fellow humans, as well as the quality of their food intake (Ames 1983). Recent research has indicated concerns that overuse of antibiotics kills beneficial bacteria in the gut, resulting in potentially permanent loss of these microbes to future generations and a plethora of health consequences (Blaser 2014). Such alteration of the gut microbiome has been linked with the rise of autoimmune and other modern ailments including allergies, asthma, diabetes, and obesity (Dai et al. 2017). Given the increasing global population, evolving living standards, food shortages, and heightened demand for animal protein production, there's a pressing need for practices to enhance agricultural and industrial productivity (Hemathilake et al. 2022). Notably, the strategic use of antibiotics in agriculture to meet the demands of a growing human populace has been associated with several advantages. Consequently, it's foreseen that nearly all animals raised and consumed for food in the future will have been exposed to some form of chemotherapy or prophylactic treatment (Lee et al. 2001).

Consumption of meats, milk, and eggs contaminated with antibiotic residues presents the concern that there can be unknowing selection of ARB and ARGs in the human gut, even when not actively undergoing antibiotic therapy. Consumption of antibiotics can favor the survival of resistant bacterial pathogens in the gut, emergence and transfer of ARGs (Pilmis et al. 2020). In the United States, EU, and many parts of the world, policies are in place, such as withholding periods, to prevent contamination of food products with antibiotic residues. Nonetheless, one recent study revealed that antibiotics can be readily detected in the feces of Chinese populations who are not undergoing any known antibiotic therapy, reinforcing the conclusion that diet is a significant source of antibiotics (Wang et al. 2020). In addition to breaches in required holding times, it is important to consider that crops grown can uptake antimicrobials that may persist in manure and other fertilizers into their edible tissues (Chitescu et al. 2013; Geng et al. 2022). Overall, the state of the knowledge presents concerns that there can be a feedback loop, providing a continuous source of exposure of human and animal gut microbes to antimicrobials via consumption of food containing antibiotic residuals as well as ARB and ARGs.

Negative Impacts of Antibiotics in Aquaculture—A Cautionary Tale

Antimicrobial residues can have negative impacts on fisheries, aquaculture, and aquatic ecosystems due to disruptions in biodiversity in ecosystem functioning in both aquaculture and wild fish. Most antibiotics used in aquaculture farms are not effectively metabolized and are often released into the surrounding environment (Gros et al. 2012). This can impact wild fish as well, especially if the water used in aquaculture environments are not effectively treated for excess antimicrobials. Even very low concentrations of antibiotics can have negative impacts on ecology. Low environmental concentrations can increase competition and more virulent disease outbreaks (Sundberg and Karvonen 2018). Shift from semi-intensive to super-intensive systems can increase fish production, but at a cost. Fish in these systems are kept in high stocking density which leads to poor water quality and disease outbreaks (Chen et al. 2014; Watts et al. 2017). Anthropogenically, this can have negative consequences as higher concentrations of residues can held within the meat of the fish even if they are wild (Watts et al. 2017). Economically, fish is a major source of animal protein and income globally, especially as human populations and corresponding demands for protein continue to grow (Agriculture Organization of the United Nations. Fisheries Department 2020; Tacon and Metian 2013). The presence of antimicrobial residues causes challenges in international trade in animal and animal products (Okocha et al. 2018). This results from the fragmentation of regulatory frameworks for the requirements of the use of antibiotics and other antimicrobials in animal husbandry.

One of the major success stories in addressing antimicrobial resistance concerns in aquaculture has been vaccination (Morrison and Saksida 2013). Specifically, the development and implementation of a vaccine against *Aeromonas salmonicida* resulted in a significant decrease in antibiotic use in the salmon industry.

Current Practices and Regulatory Frameworks Surrounding Antibiotic Use in Agriculture

The ideal approach to limit antimicrobial impacts to the environment is to limit their use in the first place. This saves cost, including cost of unnecessary use. It is much more costly to deal with the consequences of environmental contamination with antibiotics, ARB, and ARGs, than to reduce their release in the first place. However, this can be more easily said than done, and drastic measures to eliminate antibiotic use could prevent access to these life-saving drugs when they are needed. Also, without suitable alternatives in place, there could be deleterious effects on agroindustry, food availability, and cost.

Existing regulations, policies, and current practices surrounding antibiotic use vary globally, with a considerably fragmented approach. For example, in Bangladesh, laws were passed in 2010 where the use of antimicrobials, growth hormones, and pesticides were banned. The Bangladesh National Action Plan focuses on rational use, antibiotic stewardship, Good Manufacturing Practices (GMP), and comprehensive surveillance, but does not address environmental policy directly (Hoque et al. 2020). However, the operationalization and implementation of these policies remain a challenge, which is consistent with other policies that have been resented in Bangladesh and beyond (Rahman 2010). As is consistent with other Low- and Middle- Income countries (LMICs), lack of implementation or coordination, lack of financial resources, low political commitment to the policies, and building awareness of the issue are all challenges to implementing AMR policies and strategies (Hoque et al. 2020).

Comparatively, in the US, the regulatory efforts have since focused on the unnecessary usage of medically important antimicrobials, mainly held within the animal sector (Wallinga et al. 2022). Leading up to 2017, the Food and Drug Administration (FDA) worked with pharmaceutical industries to voluntarily withdraw claims on labels for the use of medically important antimicrobials in animal feeds (Center for Veterinary Medicine 2013; Sneeringer et al. 2019). This restricted growth promotion, but did not address similar doses for "disease prevention", providing a pathway for those in veterinary medicine and the agriculture sector to be able to still use antimicrobials (Spellberg et al. 2016). There are currently at least 13 medically important antimicrobials that are FDA-approved for use in feed for disease prevention with no duration limits (Wallinga et al. 2022). This allows users of these medicines to use them throughout the lifespan of the animal, as long as it can be classified as disease prevention. The implantation of these policies is also a problem in the United States because federal agencies do not collect or report farm-level use data nationally (United States Government Accountability Office 2017). Some believe that the United States has not advanced policies as much as the European Union because of a lack of political buy-in about this matter, which can cause a significant slowdown in the passing of policies (Wallinga et al. 2022).

Similar bans to those in the United States happened much earlier in the EU, and some countries, such as Denmark, responded to a voluntary call to ban antibiotic use for growth promotion in livestock as early as 1995 (Wallinga et al. 2022). Furthermore, in 2019, the European parliament voted to forbid antimicrobial use for disease prevention. Their policy is consistent with the World Health Organization's call for medically important antimicrobials for disease prevention being unnecessary and a detriment to public health, published in 2018 (Aidara-Kane et al. 2018). Under the direction of this ban, all antimicrobials that are medically important to human health should not be used to prevent disease, but medicinal antibiotics can still be used for disease treatment and control (Simjee and Ippolito 2022). Further clarifications of the appropriate use of antibiotics have been provided, citing that antibiotics have to be given on an individual animal basis and should not be given as a group treatment (Wallinga et al. 2022).

At this juncture, research into understanding how these global shifts in antibiotic use practices in agriculture impacted antibiotic residues in the environment and in food would be of great value. Of even greater value would be to be able to directly measure corresponding benefits in terms of reduced resistant infections in humans. Such studies could help to better optimize antibiotic use and practice in the future.

Knowledge Gaps and Conclusions

Antibiotics are critical life-saving drugs, and it is critical to identify practices and policies that preserve their efficacy for future generations. The more microbes are exposed to antibiotics, the more chance there is for resistant microbes to evolve, predominate, and spread. The modern era in which antibiotics are used widely in human medicine, as well as in livestock and crop production, results in continued release of antibiotics and antimicrobials to water and soil environments, orders of magnitude above natural background levels. This presents the risk that antibiotics in the environment could contribute to the evolution and spread of ARB. Antimicrobials are known to impose selective pressure on ARBs and horizontal gene transfer of ARGs, but safe discharge limits that do not contribute to the spread of antibiotic resistance have yet to be defined. Efforts are needed to define such limits in order to guide regulatory efforts and mitigation strategies. Similarly, risk assessment is needed that considers the potential of antimicrobials in the environment to contribute to the evolution and spread of antimicrobial resistance (Ashbolt et al. 2013).

In the absence of clear guidance on what is a safe level of antibiotic in the environment, if any, the ideal approach is to limit their use in the first place. This saves cost, including cost of unnecessary use. It is much more costly to deal with the consequences of environmental contamination with antibiotics, ARB, and ARGs, than to reduce their release in the first place. Great strides have been made in reducing antibiotic use in the agricultural sector, and the opportunity should be taken research the effects of this real-world experiment in microbial evolution. The emergence and spread of antimicrobial resistance in livestock and plants emphasizes the importance of addressing knowledge gaps to protect animal, environmental, and human health (Thanner et al. 2016). Critical knowledge gaps have been identified, including aspects of evolution, transmission, and interventions (Larsson et al. 2018). Contributions of different sources, including hospital and farm effluent, leakage, and other anthropogenic factors, remain understudied, as knowledge of abundance, natural variability of resistance genes, and mobilization frequencies in different types of environments are needed (Hunter et al. 2008; Larsson et al. 2018). Furthermore, a better understanding of the role of anthropogenic inputs on the evolution of antibiotic resistance is poorly understood (Bengtsson-Palme et al. 2018; Le Page et al. 2017). We also have very little understanding of the type of interventions that are effective in mitigating the emergence and spread of antibiotic spread and resistance, as evaluation of these efforts may be difficult (Ashbolt et al. 2013). One major concern with efforts to reduce antibiotic use in agriculture is to ensure that alternatives, such as vaccines, are in place. Otherwise, turning to other non-antibiotic alternatives, like heavy metals, might only act to perpetuate antibiotic resistance.

To conclude, antimicrobial residues in the environment can cause negative effects in human, animal, plant, and environmental health. Further research remains on how exactly antimicrobials residues impact the environment, but better surveillance efforts can address these issues. In addition to monitoring antimicrobials in the environment, efforts are needed to detect and monitor their impacts. Existing regulations for antimicrobials in the environment remain scattered and the extent of the implementation of these policies vary from country to country. Due to the trade of food products and the global dissemination of antimicrobials, both a worldwide and One-Health approach is needed to address antimicrobials in the environment.

References

Aga DS, Lenczewski M, Snow D, Muurinen J, Sallach JB, Wallace JS (2016) Challenges in the measurement of antibiotics and in evaluating their impacts in agroecosystems: a critical review. J Environ Qual 45. https://doi.org/10.2134/jeq2015.07.0393

Agriculture Organization of the United Nations. Fisheries Department (2020) The state of world fisheries and aquaculture. Food and Agriculture Organization of the United Nations

Aidara-Kane A, Angulo FJ, Conly JM, Minato Y, Silbergeld EK, McEwen SA, Collignon PJ, WHO Guideline Development Group Hanan Balkhy Peter Collignon John Conly Cindy Friedman Aidan Hollis Samuel Kariuki Hyo-Sun Kwak Scott McEwen Gérard Moulin Antoinette Ngandjio Bernard Rollin Flávia Rossi David Wallinga (2018) World Health Organization (WHO) guidelines on use of medically important antimicrobials in food-producing animals. Antimicrob Resist Infect Control 7:1–8

Ames BN (1983) Dietary carcinogens and anticarcinogens: oxygen radicals and degenerative diseases. Science, 221(4617):1256-1264

Aminov RI (2009) The role of antibiotics and antibiotic resistance in nature. Environ Microbiol. 2009 Dec;11(12):2970-88. Epub 2009 Jul 6. PMID: 19601960.https://doi.org/10.1111/j.1462-2920.2009.01972.x

Ashbolt NJ, Amézquita A, Backhaus T, Borriello P, Brandt KK, Collignon P, Coors A, Finley R, Gaze WH, Heberer T (2013) Human health risk assessment (HHRA) for environmental development and transfer of antibiotic resistance. Environ Health Perspect 121(9):993–1001

Bengtsson-Palme J, Larsson DGJ (2016) Concentrations of antibiotics predicted to select for resistant bacteria: proposed limits for environmental regulation. Environ Int 86:140–149

Bengtsson-Palme J, Kristiansson E, Larsson DJ (2018) Environmental factors influencing the development and spread of antibiotic resistance. FEMS Microbiol Rev 42(1):fux053

Blaser M (2014) Missing microbes. Henry Holt & Company, New York

Brown CL, Maile-Moskowitz A, Lopatkin AJ, Xia K, Logan L, Davis BC, Zhang L, Vikesland PJ, Pruden A (2024) Selection and horizontal gene transfer underlie microdiversity-level heterogeneity in resistance gene fate during wastewater treatment. Nat Commun 15:5412. https://doi.org/10.1038/s41467-024-49742-8

Center for Vetinary Medicine (2013) CVM GFI #213 new animal drugs and new animal drug combination products administered in or on medicated feed or drinking water of food-producing animals: recommendations for drug sponsors for voluntarily aligning product use conditions with GFI #209. FDA. https://www.fda.gov/regulatory-information/search-fda-guidance-documents/cvm-gfi-213-new-animal-drugs-and-new-animal-drug-combination-products-administered-or-medicated-feed

Chen Y, Zhu X, Yang Y, Han D, Jin J, Xie S (2014) Effect of dietary chitosan on growth performance, haematology, immune response, intestine morphology, intestine microbiota and disease resistance in gibel carp (C arassius auratus gibelio). Aquac Nutr 20(5):532–546

Chen C, Ray P, Knowlton KF, Pruden A, Xia K (2018) Effect of composting and soil type on dissipation of veterinary antibiotics in land-applied manures. Chemosphere 196:270–279. https://doi.org/10.1016/j.chemosphere.2017.12.161

Chitescu CL, Nicolau AI, Stolker AAM (2013) Uptake of oxytetracycline, sulfamethoxazole and ketoconazole from fertilised soils by plants. Food Additives and Contaminants: Part A, 30(6):1138-1146

Chow LM, Ghaly TM, Gillings MR (2021) A survey of sub-inhibitory concentrations of antibiotics in the environment. J Environ Sci 99. https://doi.org/10.1016/j.jes.2020.05.030

Dai D, Prussin AJ, Edwards MA, Marr LC, Pruden A, Vikesland PJ (2017) Factors shaping the human exposome in the built environment: opportunities for engineering control. Environ Sci Technol 51(14):7759–7774. https://doi.org/10.1021/acs.est.7b01097

Davis BC, Calarco J, Liguori K, Milligan EG, Brown CL, Gupta S, Harwood VJ, Pruden A, Keenum IM (2023) Recommendations for the use of metagenomics for routine monitoring of antibiotic resistance in wastewater and impacted aquatic environments. Curr Opin Environ Sci Technol 53. https://doi.org/10.1080/10643389.2023.2181620

Demain AL, Sanchez S (2009) Microbial drug discovery: 80 years of progress. J Antibiot (Tokyo). 2009 Jan;62(1):5-16. Epub 2009 Jan 9. PMID: 19132062; PMCID: PMC7094699. https://doi.org/10.1038/ja.2008.16

Forsberg KJ, Reyes A, Wang B, Selleck EM, Sommer MO, Dantas G (2012) The shared antibiotic resistome of soil bacteria and human pathogens. Science 337(6098):1107–1111

Garner E, Maile-Moskowitz AMM, Angeles LF, Flach C-F, Aga DS, Nambi I, Larsson DGJ, Bürgmann H, Zhang T, Vikesland PJ, Pruden A (2024) Metagenomic profiling of internationally sourced sewage influents and effluents yields insight into selecting targets for antibiotic resistance monitoring. Environ Sci Technol 58(37):16547–16559. https://doi.org/10.1021/acs.est.4c03726

Gelband H, Laxminarayan R (2015) Tackling antimicrobial resistance at global and local scales. Trends Microbiol. 23(9):524-6. doi:. PMID: 26338444. https://doi.org/10.1016/j.tim.2015.06.005

Geng J, Liu X, Wang J, Li S (2022) Accumulation and risk assessment of antibiotics in edible plants grown in contaminated farmlands: a review. Sci Total Environ 853:158616. https://doi.org/10.1016/j.scitotenv.2022.158616. Epub 2022 Sep 8

Grenni P, Ancona V, Caracciolo AB (2018) Ecological effects of antibiotics on natural ecosystems: A review. Microchemical J, 136:25–39

Gros M, Rodríguez-Mozaz S, Barceló D (2012) Fast and comprehensive multi-residue analysis of a broad range of human and veterinary pharmaceuticals and some of their metabolites in surface and treated waters by ultra-high-performance liquid chromatography coupled to quadrupole-linear ion trap tandem mass spectrometry. J Chromatogr A 1248:104–121

Hemamalini N, Shanmugam SA, Kathirvelpandian A, Deepak A, Kaliyamurthi V, Suresh E (2022) A critical review on the antimicrobial resistance, antibiotic residue and metagenomics-assisted antimicrobial resistance gene detection in freshwater aquaculture environment. Aquac Res 53(2):344–366. https://doi.org/10.1111/are.15601

Hemathilake DMKS, Gunathilake DMCC (2022) Agricultural productivity and food supply to meet increased demands. In Future foods (pp. 539-553). Academic Press

Hong P-Y, Al-Jassim N, Ansari MI, Mackie RI (2013) Environmental and public health implications of water reuse: antibiotics, antibiotic resistant bacteria, and antibiotic resistance genes. Antibiotics 2(3):Article 3. https://doi.org/10.3390/antibiotics2030367

Hoque R, Ahmed SM, Naher N, Islam MA, Rousham EK, Islam BZ, Hassan S (2020) Tackling antimicrobial resistance in Bangladesh: a scoping review of policy and practice in human, animal and environment sectors. PLoS One 15(1):e0227947. https://doi.org/10.1371/journal.pone.0227947

Huijbers PMC, Flach CF, Larsson DGJ (2019) A conceptual framework for the environmental surveillance of antibiotics and antibiotic resistance. Environ Int 130:104880. Epub 2019 Jun 18.PMID: 31220750. https://doi.org/10.1016/j.envint.2019.05.074

Hunter PR, Wilkinson DC, Catling LA, Barker GC (2008) Meta-analysis of experimental data concerning antimicrobial resistance gene transfer rates during conjugation. Appl Environ Microbiol 74(19):6085–6090

Jadeja NB, Worrich A (2022) From gut to mud: dissemination of antimicrobial resistance between animal and agricultural niches. Environ Microbiol 24(8):3290–3306. https://doi.org/10.1111/1462-2920.15927

Kools SA, Moltmann JF, Knacker T (2008) Estimating the use of veterinary medicines in the European union. Regul Toxicol Pharmacol. 50(1):59-65. Epub 2007 Jun 21. PMID: 18006198. https://doi.org/10.1016/j.yrtph.2007.06.003

Kristiansson E, Fick J, Janzon A, Grabic R, Rutgersson C, Weijdegård B, Söderström H, Larsson DG (2011) Pyrosequencing of antibiotic-contaminated river sediments reveals high levels of resistance and gene transfer elements. PLoS One 6(2):e17038. https://doi.org/10.1371/journal.pone.0017038. PMID: 21359229; PMCID: PMC3040208

Lamshöft M, Sukul P, Zühlke S, Spiteller M (2007) Metabolism of 14 C-labelled and non-labelled sulfadiazine after administration to pigs. Anal Bioanal Chem 388:1733–1745

Larsson DGJ, Andremont A, Bengtsson-Palme J, Brandt KK, de Roda Husman AM, Fagerstedt P, Fick J, Flach C-F, Gaze WH, Kuroda M, Kvint K, Laxminarayan R, Manaia CM, Nielsen KM, Plant L, Ploy M-C, Segovia C, Simonet P, Smalla K et al (2018) Critical knowledge gaps and research needs related to the environmental dimensions of antibiotic resistance. Environ Int 117:132–138. https://doi.org/10.1016/j.envint.2018.04.041

Larsson DG (2014) Pollution from drug manufacturing: review and perspectives. Philos Trans R Soc Lond B Biol Sci 369(1656):20130571. PMID: 25405961; PMCID: PMC4213584https://doi.org/10.1098/rstb.2013.0571

Le Page G, Gunnarsson L, Snape J, Tyler CR (2017) Integrating human and environmental health in antibiotic risk assessment: a critical analysis of protection goals, species sensitivity and antimicrobial resistance. Environ Int 109:155–169

Lee MH, Lee HJ, Ryu PD (2001) Public health risks: Chemical and antibiotic residues-review. Asian-Australasian J of Animal Sciences, 14(3):402-413

Malagón-Rojas JN, Parra Barrera EL, Lagos L (2020) From environment to clinic: the role of pesticides in antimicrobial resistance. Revista Panamericana de Salud Pública 44. https://doi.org/10.26633/RPSP.2020.44

Manz KE, Feerick A, Braun JM et al (2023) Non-targeted analysis (NTA) and suspect screening analysis (SSA): a review of examining the chemical exposome. J Expo Sci Environ Epidemiol 33:524–536. https://doi.org/10.1038/s41370-023-00574-6

Mays C, Garza GL, Waite-Cusic J, Radniecki TS, Navab-Daneshmand T (2021) Impact of biosolids amendment and wastewater effluent irrigation on enteric antibiotic-resistant bacteria – a greenhouse study. Water Res X 13:100119. https://doi.org/10.1016/j.wroa.2021.100119. PMID: 34585133; PMCID: PMC8452883

McKinney CW, Loftin KA, Meyer MT, Davis JG, Pruden A (2010) Tet and sul antibiotic resistance genes in livestock lagoons of various operation type, configuration, and antibiotic occurrence. Environ Sci Technol 44(16):6102–6109

Morrison DB, Saksida S (2013) Trends in antimicrobial use in Marine Harvest Canada farmed salmon production in British Columbia (2003–2011). The Canadian Veterinary J, 54(12):1160

Mulchandani R, Wang Y, Gilbert M, Van Boeckel TP (2023) Global trends in antimicrobial use in food-producing animals: 2020 to 2030. PLOS Global Public Health 3(2):e0001305

Murray AK, Zhang L, Yin X, Zhang T, Buckling A, Snape J, Gaze WH (2018) Novel insights into selection for antibiotic resistance in complex microbial communities. MBio 9(4):e00969–e00918. https://doi.org/10.1128/mBio.00969-18. PMID: 30042197; PMCID: PMC6058293
Okocha RC, Olatoye IO, Adedeji OB (2018) Food safety impacts of antimicrobial use and their residues in aquaculture. Public Health Rev 39(1):21. https://doi.org/10.1186/s40985-018-0099-2
Pilmis B, Le Monnier A., Zahar JR (2020) Gut microbiota, antibiotic therapy and antimicrobial resistance: a narrative review. Microorganisms, 8(2):269
Pruden A, Pei R, Storteboom H, Carlson KH (2006) Antibiotic resistance genes as emerging contaminants: studies in northern Colorado. Environ Sci Technol 40(23):7445-50. PMID: 17181002. https://doi.org/10.1021/es060413l
Rahman S (2010). OR modelling and public policies in Bangladesh: implementation challenges
Simjee S, Ippolito G (2022) European regulations on prevention use of antimicrobials from January 2022. Braz J Vet Med 44:e000822. https://doi.org/10.29374/2527-2179.bjvm000822
Sneeringer S, Bowman M, Clancy M (2019) The US and EU animal pharmaceutical industries in the age of antibiotic resistance
Spellberg B, Hansen GR, Kar A, Cordova CD, Price LB, Johnson JR (2016) Antibiotic resistance in humans and animals. NAM Perspect
Sundberg L-R, Karvonen A (2018) Minor environmental concentrations of antibiotics can modify bacterial virulence in co-infection with a non-targeted parasite. Biol Lett 14(12):20180663. https://doi.org/10.1098/rsbl.2018.0663
Tacon AG, Metian M (2013) Fish matters: importance of aquatic foods in human nutrition and global food supply. Rev Fish Sci 21(1):22–38
Thanner S, Drissner D, Walsh F (2016) Antimicrobial resistance in agriculture. MBio 7(2). https://doi.org/10.1128/mbio.02227-15
Thiele-Bruhn S, Beck IC (2005) Effects of sulfonamide and tetracycline antibiotics on soil microbial activity and microbial biomass. Chemosphere 59(4):457-65. PMID: 15788168. https://doi.org/10.1016/j.chemosphere.2005.01.023
United Nations Environment Programme (UNEP) (2023) Bracing for superbugs: strengthening environmental action in the one health response to antimicrobial resistance. ISBN: 978-92-807-4006-6
United States Government Accountability Office (2017) Antibiotic resistance: more information needed to oversee use of medically important drugs in food animals (GAO-17-192). https://www.gao.gov/assets/gao-17-192.pdf
Van Epps A, Blaney L (2016) Antibiotic residues in animal waste: occurrence and degradation in conventional agricultural waste management practices. Curr Pollut Rep 2:135–155
Wallace JS, Garner ED, Pruden A, Aga DS (2018) Occurrence and transformation of veterinary antibiotics and antibiotic resistance. Environ Pollut 15:764–772
Wallinga D, Smit LAM, Davis MF, Casey JA, Nachman KE (2022) A review of the effectiveness of current US policies on antimicrobial use in meat and poultry production. Current Environmental Health Reports 9(2):339–354. https://doi.org/10.1007/s40572-022-00351-x
Wang Q, Duan YJ, Wang SP, Wang LT, Hou ZL, Cui YX, Hou J, Das R, Mao DQ, Luo Y (2020) Occurrence and distribution of clinical and veterinary antibiotics in the faeces of a Chinese population. J Hazard Mater 383:121129. https://doi.org/10.1016/j.jhazmat.2019.121129. Epub 2019 Sep 7. PMID: 31546217
Watts JE, Schreier HJ, Lanska L, Hale MS (2017) The rising tide of antimicrobial resistance in aquaculture: sources, sinks and solutions. Mar Drugs 15(6):158
WHO (2021) WHO integrated global surveillance on ESBL-producing *E. coli* using a "one health" approach: implementation and opportunities
Wilkinson JL, Boxall ABA, Kolpin DW, Leung KMY, Lai RWS, Galbán-Malagón C, Adell AD, Mondon J, Metian M, Marchant RA, Bouzas-Monroy A, Cuni-Sanchez A, Coors A, Carriquiriborde P, Rojo M, Gordon C, Cara M, Moermond M, Luarte T, Petrosyan V, Perikhanyan Y, Mahon CS, McGurk CJ, Hofmann T, Kormoker T, Iniguez V, Guzman-Otazo J, Tavares JL, Gildasio De Figueiredo F, Razzolini MTP, Dougnon V, Gbaguidi G, Traoré O, Blais JM, Kimpe

LE, Wong M, Wong D, Ntchantcho R, Pizarro J, Ying G, Chen C, Páez M, Martínez-Lara J, Otamonga J, Poté J, Ifo SA, Wilson P, Echeverría-Sáenz S, Udikovic-Kolic N, Milakovic M, Fatta-Kassinos D, Ioannou-Ttofa L, Belušová V, Vymazal J, Cárdenas-Bustamante M, Kassa BA, Garric J, Chaumot A, Gibba P, Kunchulia I, Seidensticker S, Lyberatos G, Halldórsson HP, Melling M, Shashidhar T, Lamba M, Nastiti A, Supriatin A, Pourang N, Abedini A, Abdullah O, Gharbia SS, Pilla F, Chefetz B, Topaz T, Yao KM, Aubakirova B, Beisenova R, Olaka L, Mulu JK, Chatanga P, Ntuli V, Blama NT, Sherif S, Aris AZ, Looi LJ, Niang M, Traore ST, Oldenkamp R, Ogunbanwo O, Ashfaq M, Iqbal M, Abdeen Z, O'Dea A, Morales-Saldaña JM, Custodio M, de la Cruz H, Navarrete I, Carvalho F, Gogra AB, Koroma BM, Cerkvenik-Flajs V, Gombač M, Thwala M, Choi K, Kang H, Ladu JLC, Rico A, Amerasinghe P, Sobek A, Horlitz G, Zenker AK, King AC, Jiang J, Kariuki R, Tumbo M, Tezel U, Onay TT, Lejju JB, Vystavna Y, Vergeles Y, Heinzen H, Pérez-Parada A, Sims DB, Figy M, Good D, Teta C (2022) Pharmaceutical pollution of the world's rivers. Proc Natl Acad Sci USA 119(8):e2113947119. https://doi.org/10.1073/pnas.2113947119

Vikesland P, Garner E, Gupta S, Kang S, Maile-Moskowitz A, Zhu N (2019) Differential Drivers of Antimicrobial Resistance across the World. Acc Chem Res 52(4):916-924. Epub 2019 Mar 8. PMID: 30848890. https://doi.org/10.1021/acs.accounts.8b00643

Chapter 4
Animal Movements and Food as Driving Factors for the Spread of Antimicrobial Resistance

Benno ter Kuile, Vangelis K. Economou, Monika Dolejska, and Marisa Haenni

Abstract Antimicrobial resistance does not remain in the area where the antibiotics that selected for it were applied. Animals carrying bacteria that are resistant to antimicrobials are transported, often over relatively short distances, but also on a global scale. In addition, this transport can cause deterioration of the health of animals, resulting in infection that must be treated with antibiotics. During transport to slaughterhouses, resistant pathogens are often exchanged between animals of different batches, causing a risk for contamination of the meat with resistant bacteria. The role of wildlife in spreading of antibiotic resistance is at present poorly documented, but the available data suggest that it is very complex. Any surveillance and monitoring systems should be designed from a One-Health perspective. Considerable spreading occurs through foodstuffs, but possibly not as much as previously assumed. Resistance selected for in the livestock sector reaches human health care by a variety or routes. The resistance against critically important antimicrobials for human health care must also be viewed from the One-Health perspective. Research should prioritize understanding of the complex interactions between the various reservoirs and selection spots for antimicrobials resistance.

Keywords AMR spreading · Wildlife · Resistance selection · Animal transport · One-health · Critically important antimicrobials

---

B. ter Kuile (✉)
Department of Molecular Biology and Microbial Food Safety, Swammerdam Institute of Life Sciences, University of Amsterdam, Amsterdam, The Netherlands

Netherlands Food and Consumer Product Safety Authority, Utrecht, The Netherlands
e-mail: b.h.terkuile@uva.nl

V. K. Economou
Laboratory of Animal Food Products Hygiene – Veterinary Public Health, School of Veterinary Medicine, Aristotle University of Thessaloniki, Thessaloniki, Greece
e-mail: boikonom@vet.auth.gr

B. ter Kuile (ed.), *Antimicrobial Resistance and Antibiotics Usage in Livestock*,
https://doi.org/10.1007/978-3-032-04598-0_4

Introduction

The dissemination of antimicrobial resistance is an issue of public health importance in which various sectors and factors play their roles. Since the beginning of the antibiotic era, AMR has been increasingly reported not only in hospitals but also in livestock. Countermeasures to reduce the spread of resistance have been implemented, for example the ban on use of antibiotics as growth-promoter in the EU member states and other countries. In parallel, guidelines for prudent use have been formulated for veterinary application of antimicrobials. Increased understanding of the molecular mechanisms for development and selection of resistance have been translated into guidelines to avoid exposure to non-lethal concentrations and to treat with the highest dosage the animal can tolerate for the shortest time needed to clear the infection.

By now, the simple measures primarily aiming at reduction of use are most of the time in place, or are at the very least known in principle. Therefore, a conference was held to brainstorm about specific measures to be taken in specific situations that have the potential to further reduce selection and spread of resistance. In this chapter, the ideas are expanded on tailor-made countermeasures to prevent distribution after resistance selection has taken place, focusing on the role of animal transport, wildlife, and foodstuffs as a route. A reflection on the specifics in this respect for critically important antimicrobials rounds off the chapter.

Role of Animal Transport in Antimicrobial Resistance Transmission

Animal transport remains an important factor in the emergence of disease among animals and dissemination of several pathogenicity traits among distant areas around the globe (Sterchi et al. 2019). The transport of animals is a crucial part of

M. Dolejska
Central European Institute of Technology, University of Veterinary Sciences Brno, Brno, Czechia

Department of Biology and Wildlife Diseases, University of Veterinary Sciences Brno, Brno, Czechia

Division of Clinical Microbiology and Immunology, Department of Laboratory Medicine, The University Hospital Brno, Brno, Czechia

Faculty of Medicine in Pilsen, Charles University, Pilsen, Czechia

Department of Chemistry and Biochemistry, Faculty of AgroSciences, Mendel University in Brno, Brno, Czech Republic

M. Haenni
ANSES – Université de Lyon, Unité Antibiorésistance et Virulence Bactériennes, Lyon, France
e-mail: Marisa.HAENNI@anses.fr

the agrifood economy that has direct impact, among others, on animal production and food safety (Valadez-Noriega et al. 2018). The most common purposes include livestock movement for sale or slaughter, companion animals in terms of leisure travel or change of residence, and transport for sport activities (e.g. horses). The companion animals transport can be categorized as commercial and non-commercial, with different characteristics and legislation governing them (Tateo et al. 2022). Animal transport is regulated by appropriate legislation in most areas around the globe, with respect to the animal and production needs. Specifically, the World Organisation on Animal Health has specific provisions in chapters 7.1 to 7.3 of the Terrestrial Animal Health Code (WOAH 2023b) and in chapters 5.5 and 5.10 of the Aquatic Animal Health Code (WOAH 2023a). The European Union has established a legal framework since 1991, with the most recent being the Council Regulation (EC) No 1/2005. In the USA, the 28-hour law (United States Code, 49 U.S.C. 80,502) is in place, whereas in Canada, part XII of the Health of Animals Regulations (C.R.C., c. 296) sets rules for the animal fitness for transport. Among the animals reared in the EU in 2021 (76 million cattle, 142 million pigs, 60 million sheep, 11 million goats and billions of poultry) (ECA 2023), approximately 70% of them were transported within the EU for further production and/or slaughter. The trade with third countries represents less than 10% of the EU animal transport. Usually animals are transported through land-based vehicles, such as trucks, and to a lesser extent trains. Transportation by ship is not negligible whereas approximately 2% is carried by air (ECA 2023). The transport conditions can involve shipment in reusable containers (e.g. poultry, turkeys, rabbits) or as free roaming animals, sometimes restricted in compartments for behavioural or protection reasons (e.g. small and large ruminants, pigs and horses).

Animal Health and Transport

Animal transport is governed by strict regulations in most countries since the process is in itself stressful for the animals, because it is an unusual condition that involves fear and sometimes pain. There are several factors that influence the severity of the effects. These include animal, husbandry, and journey related factors. The perception of the animals, based on previous experience and their health condition, can influence the extent of effects. Husbandry factors are quite broad, including travel related preparations such as withdrawal of feed and water, and environmental conditions (temperature, age at transport, societal characteristics of animal breeding, etc.) (Ferguson and Warner 2008; Padalino et al. 2020). Still, the most important part is the journey itself, with factors related to the vehicle e.g. overcrowding, environmental characteristics (temperature, aeration), floor type, partitions, mixing of animals or to external factors such as driving skills, noise, vibration, road quality, and duration, being crucial. Stressors during transport can be assessed by several health indicators. It is well known, based on observations in slaughter animals, that transport can greatly affect meat quality, with meat characteristics such as pale, soft, exudative (PSE), or dark firm and dry (DFD) and increased meat spoilage being directly related to abuse during transport (Chambers et al. 2001; Ferguson and Warner 2008). Furthermore, the effects of transport include greater morbidity, mortality, live weight losses and carcass bruising (Miranda-de la Lama et al. 2014). The age of the animals is a key factor, since young animals are more vulnerable to disease. The naïve immune system along with the lack of immunity increases their susceptibility, as shown by immunosuppression in lambs and increased rates of bovine respiratory disease cases in calves that have been associated with travel (Miranda-de la Lama et al. 2014). Morbidity during transport also transpires, with more than 70% of the deaths occurring on the truck and 30% at the slaughterhouse, with death usually related to younger animals. The weight loss observed is related to stressors and the water/feed deprivation prior to transport that is exercised in some animal types, with young animals being less prone to the effect than older ones (Fisher et al. 2009).

Companion animals also experience travel as a stressful activity. Travel influences the physiological and emotional state of the animals *via* specific effects on their physiology and metabolism (Tateo et al. 2022). Factors such as prolonged fasting periods, restricted space and the poorly constructed containers add to the discomfort. The immediate deprivation of the daily routine of the animal as summarized in lack of stimuli, separation from familiar animals, isolation and previous bad travel experiences, can affect the proper behaviour of dogs and cats (Tateo et al. 2022). As a result, severe anxiety and suffering will emerge, as exhibited by barking, over-excitement, vomiting, and phobias (Tateo et al. 2022). In addition, the transport of companion animals for sports, recreation, and scientific research is also increasing. The effect on dogs is reported to activate the hypothalamus–pituitary–adrenal axis, leading to release of catecholamines and glucocorticoids, and consequent haematological responses (neutrophil increase and lymphocyte decrease). Even short car transports lasting 50 minutes can induce an effect on acute stress markers in dogs (Chmelikova et al. 2020; Tateo et al. 2022). Cats are reported to be prone to travel discomfort; however, little scientific data exist (Tateo et al. 2022). Horses are reported to exhibit balance disorders and stress exhibited with gastrointestinal deficiencies, decreased gastrointestinal sounds and gastric ulceration post transportation (Padalino and Raidal 2020).

Transport Conditions that Can Facilitate AMR Dissemination

Animal transport has concerned the public mainly in terms of animal welfare and its importance as a branch of the production chain; however, the involvement of animal movement, as human induced transport or migration, has been extensively linked to pathogen spread (Fevre et al. 2006). Transport by itself can be considered a part of the concentrated animal feeding operations that have been characterized as a source of antibiotic-resistant pathogenic bacteria, with exposures of humans being documented via multiple pathways. Recent reports suggest that international travel may play a greater role than previously thought, suggesting that geographic trends in AMR may be more important than national antimicrobial use (Frost et al. 2019). There are scarce reports of the small yet higher risk of carriage in the dissemination of AMR by companion animals (Guardabassi et al. 2004; Jin et al. 2012; Meyer et al. 2012). However, little information is available regarding the role of companion animals in travel-induced AMR spread and the factors influencing it. While the effects of companion animal travel are expected to be similar to those of production animals, actual data remain scarce.

The effects of transport on the animals are characterized as a rather stressful process, leading to increased pathogen dissemination and AMR occurrence. Specifically, poultry transportation to farms or abattoirs involves noise, manual or mechanic catching, loading into crates or cages, high stocking densities and feed and water withdrawal; all these can be rather aggravating conditions. Poultry farming also requires several stages until slaughter (elite, grandparent flocks, hatchery etc.) with transport being rather frequent and performed in reusable crates that further enhances pathogen transmission. Male calves of dairy breeds are usually moved to fattening farms, a process that is related to adverse health effects and increased AMR carriage (Gay et al. 2019). These animals are frequently treated with antimicrobials on arrival (Bouma and Lenski 1988; Jarrige et al. 2017), a practice that is probably related to higher AMR Levels in bacteria from calves (Tenhagen et al. 2018). Pig transport is mostly for slaughter or reproduction since in several cases the animals are reared in the same farm that they were born. The shipments to abattoirs are therefore the most common form of pig transport (Crescio et al. 2021).

Generally, the transport practices that affect AMR occurrence involve AMU before shipping or on arrival, as reported for certain animal species (Padalino et al. 2016; Cirone et al. 2019; Pratelli et al. 2021; Nicolaisen et al. 2023) and the immune readiness of the animal during transport as exhibited by stress and health effects, that are reported to relate greatly to journey duration (Nielsen et al. 2011). Concerning the possible human/animal interactions, it is reported specifically for cattle that transport personnel and their interactions with the animals are quite important in the entire transport process from the initial preparation, the loading, the transport, to the delivery of the animals to the destination (Nicolaisen et al. 2023).

AMR Contamination Through Transport

The movement of animals can spread infectious agents between farms or from farms to other destinations, e.g. slaughterhouses. Specifically, for production animals, younger animals are usually transported; therefore, the effect on pathogen carriage is prolonged to larger time periods and helps the spread to a multitude of locations in a global level. Furthermore, the possible health effects require therapy with antibiotics that can select the antibiotic resistant bacteria or antibiotic resistance genes (ARBs/ARGs) within the gastrointestinal tract of these animals (Anjum et al. 2019). The well-established routes of contamination involve water (used for irrigation, contaminated by manure/used for agricultural produce), animal products and surface sources. Recently, ARBs/ARGs have been recognized as possible vectors that can be transmitted through air (Zhao et al. 2022). Concerning the load of ARBs/ARGs on animals, their transmission can be direct through contact with other animals or indirect through water, feed, surfaces, fomites and airborne transmission. The animals can themselves contaminate the environment through excretions (*via* urine, faeces, vomit or saliva), a route that can be quite problematic if the disinfection procedures are not effective, with the concentration of ARBs/ARGs on the animal's excrements being rather important. The dispersal of these infectious material through the fast-moving vehicles is a procedure that has not been extensively researched in is of great importance to the dispersal of them along the travel route.

Specific characteristics of transport conditions that influence ABRs/ARGs proliferation are, among others, feed and water withdrawal, occurrence of possible additional stressors, general health status of the animals and environmental conditions of the travel. Feed and water withdrawal effect depends on the animals transported; in pigs it is a common practice resulting to better hygiene of the carcass. However, there are potential negative effects related to prolonged starvation (Martin-Pelaez et al. 2009) resulting in microbiome disturbance (Massacci et al. 2020) and favouring increased shedding of possibly AMR enteric bacteria, such as *Salmonella* (Verbrugghe et al. 2011), or increased mobilization of plasmids (Guiney et al. 1995). In poultry it increases the caecal and crop prevalence and shedding of *Salmonella* spp. and *Campylobacter* spp. (Joat et al. 2021), bacteria that frequently harbour ARGs. However, feed restriction in countries with higher temperatures has been associated with lesser impact of heat stress (Tsiouris et al. 2014). In calves, feed and water withdrawal causes increased gut permeability (Pisoni et al. 2022) and diarrhoea (Araujo et al. 2015), leading to increased cross-contamination between animals and the environment. In cattle and sheep destined for slaughter, prolonged feed withdrawal is associated with increased multiplication of *Salmonella* spp. and *E. coli* (Cray Jr. et al. 1998). Stressors during transport can trigger the hypothalamic–pituitary–adrenal activity and the release of various stress hormones, leading to gut/blood barrier disruption and proliferation of enteric pathogens. The stressors relate to the release of catecholamines and adrenaline which are usually triggered by harsh treatment or just by adverse transport conditions (increased temperature, inappropriate space or mixing of animals from different species or origin) (Valkova et al. 2022). Still, little information is available specifically for transport stressors and AMR dissemination. Specifically, though, certain environmental conditions, such as increased temperature and humidity, can have direct effect on the proliferation of the respiratory and intestinal microbiota. ARBs or pathogens possibly residing in the animal's body can multiply faster at higher temperatures and therefore can easily contaminate surfaces, animals, or humans. Lastly, the health status of the animal prior to transport is of importance; sick animals should not be transported for a variety of reasons. Hence if transport occurs, the possibility of ARBs/ARGs transmission increases because of poor immune system condition, pathogen occurrence or AMU prior to transport. Still, this is another area that has not been investigated extensively.

During transport, the shedding of bacteria from the animals is highly possible, augmenting the risk of transmission by direct contamination of other animals or through surfaces. Specifically, the higher rate of fecal oral contamination has been proven for *Salmonella* and *Campylobacter* in pigs and poultry. Transmission through ingestion has been also considered for extended-spectrum beta-lactamase (ESBL) and carbapenem-resistant Enterobacterales (CRE), as well as for *Clostridioides difficile* (Manaia 2017). Further, the inadequate cleaning and disinfecting of the vehicle can worsen the contamination and further disperse the ARBs/ARGs present. The most important excretion in terms of contamination are feces, even though other biological material, such as urine, saliva and milk, can also contribute. Specifically, fecal microbial contamination depends on the fecal volume and their microbial load, with factors such as the ingested feed, intestinal motility, stressors, and the carriage of ABRs/ARGs by the animals. It has been shown that hide contamination is highly dependent on the transport conditions, an observation possibly linked to the increased defecation, as reported in cattle hides for *Salmonella* spp. (Dewell et al. 2008) and *E. coli* O157 (Arthur et al. 2010). Still direct contact should not be underestimated, since it involves ARBs of the urogenital tract such as vancomycin-resistant enterococci (VRE), ESBL and CRE or the skin including ESBL, CRE and methicillin-resistant *Staphylococcus aureus* (MRSA).

It seems that the duration of the transport is of importance by itself, resulting in prolonged contact between animals, feed withdrawal for longer periods and impairment of the immune system (Schwartzkopf-Genswein et al. 2012). Longer journey has been associated with higher contamination of cattle hides with *Salmonella* spp. and *E. coli* O157 (Dewell et al. 2008). Further, transport to slaughterhouses can vary from short distance travel to larger distances, often involving multiple countries. Regardless of the duration, stress related factors include animal welfare as affected by the husbandry system and health status of animals, and their arrival at the slaughterhouse environment, which is quite stressful to the animals and can be largely affected by personnel (Nicolaisen et al. 2023).

The transport environment can also be a vector of ARBs/ARGs with which the animals can come in contact. Cleaning and disinfection of trucks and control posts after animal transport is advised or, as in the EU, obligatory (Council Regulation No 1/2005). Nevertheless, the area and surfaces can remain contaminated by pathogens such as *Salmonella* (Magistrali et al. 2008) and other Enterobacterales (Mannion et al. 2008), thus exposing animals to ARB/ARGs during the transport. Specifically, Magistrali et al. reported that *Salmonella* spp. isolates from pig carcasses were different from the ones found in the animals in the farm of origin, therefore implying contamination during travel (Magistrali et al. 2008). A similar observation has been made for MRSA (Broens et al. 2011). In poultry, the hygiene of the crates is a major issue, with several studies reporting the occurrence of *Salmonella* and ARBs on these crates, interestingly in higher counts after cleaning than before (Zeng et al. 2021). Several ARBs have been detected in the crates, including MDR bacteria such as *A. baumannii*, *K. pneumoniae*, ESBL-producing *E. coli*, colistin-resistant *E. coli* and VRE (von Tippelskirch et al. 2018; Molechan et al. 2019; McIver et al. 2020; Savin et al. 2020).

Airborne transmission during transport has been reported for aerosol particles carrying ARB, with factors such as contact proximity and the survival of the ARB in the environment being of importance. The main ARBs transmitted by inhalation include bacteria affecting the respiratory system (MRSA, VRE, ESBL and CRE) (Manaia 2017). Antibiotic resistant enterococci have been isolated from air and surface samples of vehicles (Rule et al. 2008). Dust particles can also permit survival of bacteria that otherwise would not survive the environmental conditions, e.g. ARBs such as *E. coli* (Nguyen et al. 2022). This is particularly important for dried fecal material, as shown in the transmission via dried fecal dust of MRSA (Schmithausen et al. 2018), VRE (Novais et al. 2013), and ESBL-producing Enterobacteriaceae (Davies and Wales 2019). Generally, transport vehicles are considered to disseminate contaminants to a variable yet higher degree. Specifically, fast moving objects like the ones used to transport animals, tend to disperse airborne or bioaerosol related particles in higher rates than static animal gatherings and buildings. The prediction and quantification of dispersal is quite difficult since specific models should be constructed. In addition, several variables need to be considered. These include the environmental stability of the factors and therefore their survival, the possibility of airborne transmission, the landscape and topology of the area of travel, the animal species transported, and the density and distance of animal as well as human activities close to transport routes or destination points (Münch et al. 2017).

The Role of Wild Animal Movements in Transmission of Antimicrobial Resistance

Resistant microbes selected by antibiotic use in the human and agriculture sectors subsequently spread to the environment and reached wildlife living in human-influenced habitats. AMR was observed in various species of wild animals around the globe, which were proved to carry MDR high-risk human clones as well as genes conferring resistances to last-line antibiotics, such as carbapenems or colistin (Dolejska and Papagiannitsis 2018; Ben Yahia et al. 2020; Loucif et al. 2022; Wink et al. 2022; Wyrsch et al. 2022; Ahlstrom et al. 2023a, b). Although many studies documented the dissemination of MDR bacteria into wildlife, they also raised important gaps in our understanding of the role of wild animal species in the complex transmission pathways of AMR. Most of these studies focused on wildlife as sentinels affected by anthropogenic activities and showing the level of environmental contamination by AMR (Dolejska and Literak 2019; Ramey and Ahlstrom 2020), but fewer studies aimed to examine wildlife as vectors or even amplifiers of AMR (Bonnedahl et al. 2015; Mathys et al. 2017; Cao et al. 2020; Ahlstrom et al. 2021a, b; Martin-Velez et al. 2024).

Sources of AMR in Wildlife

The occurrence of AMR in wildlife is a complex problem influenced by various biological, ecological and geographical factors which are not yet fully understood. Urbanization greatly influences breeding and feeding habits of certain wildlife species, creating connections between wildlife and humans and supporting the cross-transmission of AMR. Although assigning the source and directionality of AMR dissemination is challenging, several transmission routes of AMR to wildlife have been suggested (Fig. 4.1). Wild animals inhabiting human-influenced environments can easily acquire ARBs from urban waste. Wastewater treatment plants (WWTP) processing sewage sludge from hospitals, cities and slaughterhouses are not fully efficient in removing antibiotics, disinfectants and resistant microbes. ARBs/ ARGs are thus released into surface waters (Liguori et al. 2022), and can further colonize freshwater and marine wildlife. Several studies demonstrated the links between WWTP and AMR in wildlife. Higher loads of AMR were observed in wild ducks foraging at WWTP compared to wild birds from remote areas not in contact with sewage systems (Marcelino et al. 2019). Other studies demonstrated similar genomic profiles of antibiotic resistant *E. coli* from birds and rodents with those from WWTP and hospitalized patients (Nelson et al. 2008; Guenther et al. 2013; Hansen et al. 2016; Atterby et al. 2017). In regions with poor sanitation and wastewater management the transmission of AMR into the environment can be expected to be much higher compared to high-income countries, but few investigations in wildlife from these areas have been conducted so far (Hasan et al. 2014; Ben Yahia et al. 2020). Another important source of AMR for wildlife is landfills and garbage in urban areas. A direct connection between landfill use and the occurrence of AMR was demonstrated in gulls using GPS tracking (Ahlstrom et al. 2019, 2021a, b) and highly similar CPE were found in gulls foraging in landfills and those circulating in a nearby hospital. Landfills have severe implications for wildlife as some populations switch from a natural diet to easily accessible food available in landfills, especially during low food availability in winter or high energetic demand in breeding seasons. Such a shift in feeding behaviors was observed for some populations of gulls, rooks, storks, raptors, small rodents and foxes (Plaza and Lambertucci 2017; Dolejska and Literak 2019). The source of artificial diet, coupled with climate changes, results in modifications of animal movements, such as the reduction of the home range or stopping the winter migration in some populations, and thus influences the transmission of microbes including AMR. Livestock and agriculture represent other important sources as wild animals can get into contact with livestock-associated AMR when searching for food at manured farmlands or farm environments. The analysis of small rodents captured at farms or in close vicinity showed they more often carried AMR microbes than animals from livestock-free locations (Kozak et al. 2009).

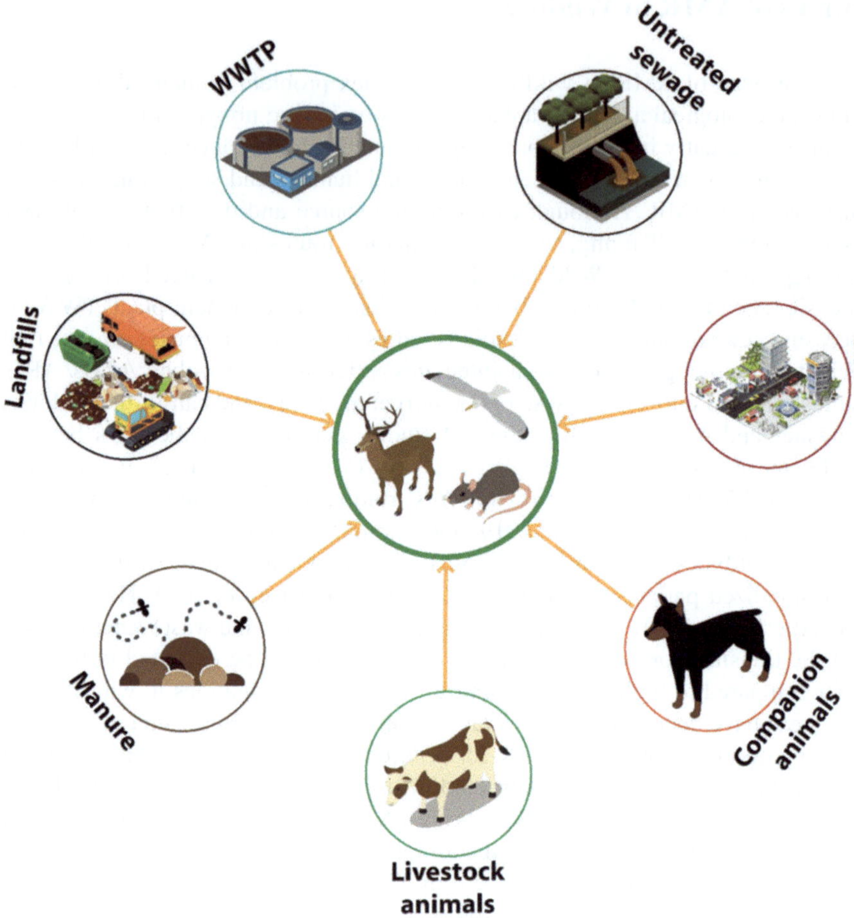

Fig. 4.1 Main source of AMR for wildlife

Wild Animals as Reservoirs and Vectors of AMR

Although wildlife is probably not a main transmission route of AMR, it represents an important pathway of resistant microbes in the environment (Fig. 4.2). As wildlife can move freely and their feces can be found anywhere, we can expect they can also further spread resistant microbes present in their gut. Wild animals associated with livestock can spread AMR between herds or outside farms, while in some regions small rodents and insects present in food processing facilities can contaminate food (Chandrakar et al. 2022; Qian et al. 2023). Gulls visiting waste sites were reported to disperse resistant microbes in the beach landscape (Simoes et al. 2010). However, it is difficult to estimate how often this direction of transmission from wildlife to the environment and from there to humans and animals actually occurs. To analyze the transmission rate, we need to know the abundance of AMR in the gut

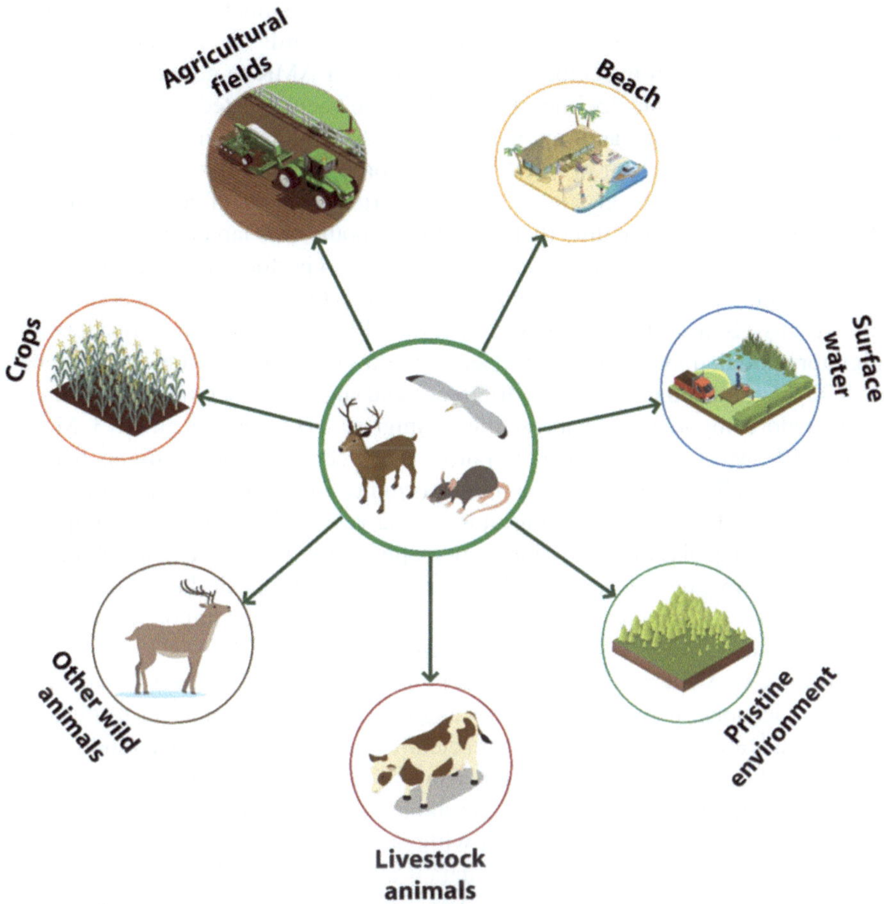

Fig. 4.2 Selected transmission pathways of AMR from wildlife

microbiota and for how long resistant microbes can persist there. Not much research has been done on these topics for wildlife so far. Moreover, separate animal populations within a specific species can vary in feeding and habitat use, resulting in different exposure to sources of AMR which makes these calculations very difficult to make and usually also impossible to generalize. A few experimental studies on the duration of shedding showed that resistant *E. coli* can be maintained in the gut of wild birds for around one month (Sandegren et al. 2018; Franklin et al. 2020), giving plenty of opportunities for further transmission. They also demonstrated frequent transfers of AMR between individuals within a flock, highlighting the importance of animals breeding in large colonies. Another important question in AMR transmission that research on wildlife has not yet answered is the level of horizontal gene transfer (HGT) of AMR within the animal gut. HGT was demonstrated as an important route of AMR dissemination in humans and farm animals, so we can assume that it also frequently happens in wildlife guts.

Information on length of shedding is also crucial for estimating the AMR transfer during seasonal migration of wildlife, especially wild birds. *Via* migration, resistant bacteria can spread from regions with high level of AMR to countries will lower AMR prevalence. Clinically important ARBs have been detected in migratory birds in remote areas with low anthropogenic impact, suggesting the importance of long-distance animal movement in AMR transmission (Guenther et al. 2017). Although migratory birds have been suggested as important vectors of resistant microbes across the globe, research directly testing this hypothesis is largely missing, mainly because such interdisciplinary studies are difficult to perform and even more difficult to design. Moreover, research conducted on this topic so far provides contradictory results. Some studies showed marked differences between resident and migratory populations of the same species in terms of AMR occurrence (Bonnedahl et al. 2015), while others found no difference and suggested that local acquisition of AMR is more important than spread during migration (Loncaric et al. 2013; Mathys et al. 2017). Most long-distance migrants make a series of shorter flights between stopover sites. These sites provide the opportunity for close interaction of species that are normally separated during most of the year and may represent important hotspots of transmission. Some innovative approaches using telemetry along with genomic profiling of resistant microbes was done in gulls on Alaska (Ahlstrom et al. 2019, 2021a, b). Such interdisciplinary research may bring us important insights in the complexity of AMR pathways in wildlife.

The topic of AMR in wildlife is too complex to be tackled as a whole. To answer the key questions, it is essential to focus our research and financial resources to targeted and tailored studies with clear scientific questions rather than random sampling of wild animals and simple reporting of ARBs/ARGs. Most of the studies published so far are one-off surveys that did not aim to identify the source of AMR and that were done in one-time point without any longitudinal observation. Most research was done in Europe and little data is available from low-income countries, providing skewed results. We already know that AMR is present in wildlife and when we search for it we will most likely find it everywhere although in different proportions. What we should aim for is the assessment of risks for humans and food animals posed by wildlife in terms of AMR transfer. However, our knowledge gaps limit our ability to estimate these risk at the moment.

As a lot of research has been done so far on AMR in wildlife, do we need surveillance system for this sector? To set up an efficient monitoring, we first need to know what species to focus on, which in the case of wildlife is much more complicated than for other sectors. Wild animals include diverse species from avian, mammal, reptiles and invertebrate families occupying land, air or water, species that are either wild, peridomestic or livestock-related, populations with local and intercontinental movement, populations in pristine areas or those in highly impacted anthropogenic regions or even wildlife such as game that we directly consume. It may not be possible to build a functioning surveillance for wildlife due to the above-mentioned complexities and existing variables. On the other hand, instead of extensive global surveillance, well-designed studies would be more valuable, performed in focal areas with described interfaces, where humans, domestic animals and the environment including wildlife closely interact. In such settings, the transmission pathways are easier to follow. The current knowledge gaps can be filled by studies respecting the One Health concept and with clear links between the human, animal and environmental parts. These investigations should be based on extensive sampling, longitudinal observations and deep molecular analysis of ARBs/ARGs (Nesporova et al. 2024). Coordination with ongoing programs of wildlife monitoring (e.g. for avian influenza) could save financial resources for field work and sampling. Also, cooperation between countries through which a given animal species passes, or in which it settles down for a certain period of time, would be of great added value.

Methods Used in AMR Research and Surveillance in Wildlife

Another important point in AMR surveillance in wildlife is the selection of appropriate target bacteria and methodology. Should we follow the monitoring pipelines established in humans, livestock and the food sector, such as focusing on EuSCAPE microbes, WHO priority pathogens and clinically important resistances (ESBL, carbapenemases, etc.)? For the comparison of wildlife results to the human and veterinary sectors, this approach would be the most appropriate. It has been proposed that *E. coli* is a good indicator of anthropogenic impact on the environment and would be a suitable indicator species for a One Health monitoring, including surface and wastewaters as well as wildlife (Anjum et al. 2021). Culture-based methods for quantifying and isolating *E. coli* are inexpensive and simple to conduct, ensuring their applicability across the globe. Selective cultivation using antibiotic-supplemented media has been extensively used to explore the occurrence of ARBs in wildlife and may be better for selection of isolates with target resistance mechanisms than cultivation without antibiotics. Methods for characterization of *E. coli* such as serotyping and multi-locus sequence typing are also available and allow easy comparison of environmental and wildlife isolates to human and animal isolates. However, such comparisons at the level of sequence type (ST) are not discriminatory enough as strains from the same ST may significantly differ at a genomic level (Jamborova et al. 2018). The outcome does not help us to follow transmission pathways and their directions. On the other hand, whole genome sequencing (WGS) gives far more information, including not only STs but also phylogenetic relationships between the strains based on the level of single-nucleotide polymorphism, the content and genetic context of ARGs, and linkage of ARGs with mobile genetic elements. WGS allows precise identification of shared bacterial strains, plasmids and their transmission between compartments (Djordjevic et al. 2024). WGS of wildlife isolates, along with comparison of publicly available bacterial genomes of human and livestock origin (e.g. Enterobase), has been successfully used in the past decade in wildlife studies (Nesporova et al. 2020; Ahlstrom et al. 2023a, b). However, fewer studies sequenced isolates directly collected from these different sectors in the studied location (Ahlstrom et al. 2021a, b; Nesporova et al.

2024). Nevertheless, genotyping of single isolates allows us to see only a small portion of the bacteria and AMR circulating in the environment and wildlife. Other methods, such as quantitative detection of selected ARGs or metagenomics approach, would provide another level of information on wildlife resistome and plasmidome, including the abundance and diversity of AMR and plasmids, thereby opening the path to risk assessment studies. Combining selection-based approaches with these cultivation-independent techniques may give us a more comprehensive picture on AMR transmission in the environment (Ahlstrom et al. 2023a, b; Lin et al. 2023).

The Role of Food in Transmission of Antimicrobial Resistance

Development and spreading of AMR is driven by a complex set of factors that interact with each other (Vikesland et al. 2019). Food, specifically raw food, is one of the exposure routes for humans (Larsson and Flach 2022). Despite ample evidence that transmission of AMR from the agricultural sector to human health care occurs, few reliable estimates exist on the attribution of the resistance encountered in human pathogens originating from food. One study on a vast dataset that succeeded in attributing ESBL exposure in humans to various sources, estimating the contribution of food at approximately 20% (Mughini-Gras et al. 2019), while another European study found very limited similarities between ESBL-producing *E. coli* and *K. pneumoniae* retrieved either from food items or clinical samples. In general, this attribution is difficult to make as it requires precise monitoring of AMR on the several potential transmission routes.

More comprehensive understanding of the dynamics of AMR within and between the various ecosystems requires a "farm-to-fork" and "One Health" approach (EFSA 2021). Within this framework, quantitative assessments of the impact of each of the major driving factors are essential to estimate the attribution of food production and the subsequent dissemination routes (Leger et al. 2021). On a global scale exposure of microbes to non-lethal concentrations of antibiotics has been identified as a key risk factor (Ter Kuile et al. 2016; Llewelyn et al. 2017). On a practical level, the translation of this general principle into practical measures that reduce selection of resistance, is complicated. The transmission of resistance via environmental routes is poorly documented and hence it is hard to predict the effect of measures aiming at reduction of AMR spreading (Lima et al. 2020a, b).

The presence or absence of ARBs on foodstuffs depend on several factors: application of antibiotics; the way antibiotics are disposed of or dispersed on a production facility afterwards; the location of farms and the way they are embedded in society; economic factors that force farmers to use undesirable production practices; consumer demands, which can be detrimental if cheap meat is demanded or beneficial if antibiotic-free food is preferred. These factors are part of a much larger societal system, that can be divided into seven themes, each containing several comparable driving factors (Lambraki et al. 2022). When searching for opportunities to reduce selection for resistance, the agricultural sector is an obvious point of focus, as animal production already takes place in a highly controlled environment that is subject to precise regulation in most countries.

One of the production related factors is hygiene in the animal living spaces (McEwen and Collignon 2018). In particular in low- and middle-income countries, lack of hygiene in the production facilities may be an important contributing factor to development and spreading of AMR (Allel et al. 2023). The EU Regulation 2019/6 provides the food safety authorities of the EU member states with enforcement tools to demand proper hygiene in animal facilities. In other countries farm hygiene may be harder to enforce. The analysis of the resistomes in the chicken gut showed the importance of good quality feed in limiting the spread of AMR microbes (Koorakula et al. 2022). Slaughterhouses form a distribution reservoir for antimicrobial resistance genes, emphasizing once more the importance of hygiene in food production facilities (Alvarez-Molina et al. 2023). Another factor is the human-animal contact. In industrialized countries this is mostly strictly controlled and transfer of microbes is limited by a set of measures, for example obligatory showers before and after entering facilities such as chicken coops or piggeries. In low and middle income countries, farm workers and workers in urban markets were often exposed to animals in a way that transfer of bacteria is highly likely (Alam et al. 2019).

Both pathogenic zoonotic bacteria and commensal bacteria from animal origin can be resistant to antibiotics. The pathogenic AMR microbes may cause more prolonged infections and more frequent treatment failure than the susceptible variants (Antunes et al. 2020). Commensal bacteria of animal origin can function as reservoirs of transferable ARGs that end up in opportunistic infectious bacteria or are transferred to pathogens inside the host. Biofilm formation facilitates the transfer of ARGs from harmless microorganisms to pathogens (Patil et al. 2021). In Tunisia, AMR and virulence were shown to correlate as the combination offered a selective evolutionary advantage to the pathogens investigated (Hassena et al. 2022). A similar co-occurrence of resistance and virulence was observed in the seafood pathogen *Aeromonas* spp. (De Silva et al. 2021).

It is uncertain whether there are specific risk products for the spreading of AMR, in the sense that resistant variants have a disproportionally higher chance of being present on a specific foodstuff than the susceptible counterpart. To identify such AMR-risk products a metagenomics-based surveillance might in the future be developed into an instrument for comparing resistomes between different collections of foodstuffs (Duarte et al. 2020). Some products may be characterized as high-AMR risk, but it is not certain that the presence of AMR exceeds the expected level based on the presence of the bacterial load. For example, milk is pinpointed as a high-risk product for MRSA (Titouche et al. 2022), however, milk always contain considerable numbers of *S. aureus*. Therefore, it cannot easily be ascertained that the chance of MRSA is disproportional. Salads and ready-to-eat food sold as street foods can be contaminated with ARBs (Giri et al. 2021). It is again not known whether the prevalence of the resistant bacteria exceeds the number estimated based on the occurrence of the susceptible equivalent. An exception may be cultured shrimp and fish, in the sense that compared to wild-caught shrimp, aquaculture shrimp had a higher prevalence of ARGs in their gut (Sharma et al. 2021).

In the framework of the spreading of resistance genes, two situations should be discerned: (1) Patients have foodborne infections with resistant bacteria or (2) the resistance genes of commensal microbes are transferred inside the gut of a consumer. The latter transfer can be plasmid-mediated or occur by means of other mobile genetic elements and HGT events (Partridge et al. 2018). The first case has direct consequences for the patient, as the cost of treatment, in additional patient suffering and financial, increases (Pulingam et al. 2022). In the human gut microbiome horizontal transfer of ARGs frequently occurs (McInnes et al. 2020). As a consequence the opportunistic pathogenic *E. coli* variants can become resistant to the antibiotics of choice, increasing health care costs (Sora et al. 2021). At the moment there is insufficient information to quantify both mechanisms and compare them with respect to costs.

Spreading of Resistance Against Critically Important Antimicrobials

Both for the human (WHO 2016) and for the veterinary sector (OIE 2015) a list of critically important antimicrobials (CIA) has been drawn up. Unfortunately there is considerable overlap between antibiotic usage in these two sectors (McEwen and Collignon 2018). Resistance selected in the veterinary sector can end up in the human health care via various routes, including food (Pires et al. 2018). Hence, it is imperative to adjust the veterinary application of CIA for human health care. When, however, such usage is unavoidable for animal health and welfare reasons, these CIA should be applied in such a manner that selection for resistance is minimal. This can only be achieved by an integrative approach, using several measures in parallel.

While the lists of CIA's used by various governments for human usage are all derived from the WHO list (WHO 2016) and differ only on minor details, the lists being used by these countries on veterinary CIA's differ considerably (Scott et al. 2019). To harmonize the definition of veterinary CIA's, these should be considered in the framework of human versus animal health, for the expected selection of resistance and for the type infections to be treated. The size and management of pig farms strongly influence the chance of resistance of faecal *E. coli* against CIA's (Lunha et al. 2020), illustrating the influence of holding practices. Such variations due to farming methods are observed for all livestock. In addition, resistance against CIA's can be selected for if bacteria resistant to several antibiotics, including a CIA, are treated by a unlisted antibiotic. The CIA resistance can then be selected for indirectly.

The volume of antimicrobials used in the care of livestock is monitored systematically in the EU (EMA 2023) and also about the rest of the world data are available (Mulchandani et al. 2023). To understand the driving factors for the usage of CIA's monitoring should specifically address these compounds and also the reasons for the choice of these antibiotics over less contested alternatives should be understood. Both sectors should develop best practices to avoid using CIA's. Voluntary cooperation with private sector partners can achieve remarkable results, shown in Canada where not using ceftiofur for a few years produced a remarkable decline in resistance against this antibiotic (Canadian 2009). In the Netherlands such decrease of resistance after reduction of antibiotic usage was observed across all types of antimicrobials applied (Veldman et al. 2023).

The most effective way to prevent development of resistance is to prevent exposure of bacteria to antimicrobials. This can be done by improving water and feed quality and by enhanced sanitation of livestock living quarters including better infrastructure (Zinsstag et al. 2023). In addition, effective measures must be identified by assessing the risks of existing environmental hazards and evolving threats. Risks can be correlated to the amounts of antibiotics that are used to neutralise their effects, thereby in fact prioritizing the hazards to be addressed. This type of measures are not restricted to use of CIA's, but are more urgent than for CIA's than for antibiotics not used by humans. A study comparing free-range and conventional poultry production demonstrated the importance of biosecurity in preventing antibiotic use (McMullin 2022). Sharing experiences with methods to reduce antimicrobial usage can be very beneficial for all parties involved (Picot et al. 2017).

Effective measures to reduce use of CIA's can only be designed in a One-Health framework that takes into account all aspects of infection prevention and treatment. Further research is needed to gain better insight in the practical feasibility of farm level measures and their acceptability for farmers. The behaviour and driving motives of farmers and veterinarians need to be understood. Full comprehension of the economic aspects of the process will allow policy makers to support their decisions with convincing information. All-in-all this type of insight will improve both the decisions and their acceptability for all partners.

Research Priorities

The importance of the transport or movement of animals in the dissemination of ARBs is disputed, and further research is needed to clarify it. Still, there is evidence supporting this possibility of large-scale dissemination; the hospital related VRE found in Europe, Asia, South America and the USA are part of a single clonal lineage suggesting common routes of dissemination among humans, livestock and animal products (Frost et al. 2019). Livestock-associated MRSA are regarded as emerging human pathogens, having a clear zoonotic character (Anjum et al. 2019). Concerning the possibility of AMR exchange between domestic and wild animals, reports are controversial. Despite the widespread opinion that AMR in wild animals depends on anthropogenic activities, there are specific AMR characters associated with the degree of human presence, while others appear to circulate in wildlife, therefore showing that wildlife AMR is not solely reliant on anthropogenic activities (Swift et al. 2019). Transport of animals can perhaps contribute to the wildlife contamination; further research on this route of contamination is needed, since these scenarios have been superficially investigated. Therefore, it is evident that the circulation of ARBs/ARGs exist in the human/animal/environment interface, to an extent that is yet to be calculated.

Across the board, there is considerable information on the prevalence of resistant bacteria on the unprocessed products at the source of the various food production chains (EFSA 2021). To track ARBs/ARGs through the food chain, quantitative attribution at each stage is needed, supported by genetic analysis, a consideration that also applies to ARBs/ARGs in wildlife. The attribution of various sources to resistance in human health care is under dispute (Antimicrobial Resistance 2022). If ESBL data (Mughini-Gras et al. 2019) are extrapolated to overall resistance, selection in agriculture may account for one-fifth to one-quarter of resistance in human pathogens. However, resistant bacteria can reach humans through several routes other than animal products (Blaak et al. 2015a, b), and given that most antibiotics are used in livestock rather than humans (Dadgostar 2019), the total selective pressure from agriculture is likely much greater than gene transfer through food alone would suggest. For these reasons documenting AMR transfer necessitates consideration of epidemiology at the plasmid level, particularly given the major role played by HGT and the possible plasmid changes it can induce (Bengtsson-Palme et al. 2018). Moreover, the dose-response relationship (the level of ARB contamination in food required to cause a corresponding incidence of resistance in the human host) is not known. Quantitative microbial risk assessment, supplemented by modern molecular methods, can help estimate the prevalence of ARBs on food and the associated risk of transfer to the human population (Haas 2020), therefore enhancing the effectiveness of risk reduction efforts.

Acknowledgements The project was partially supported by the Grant 2024ITA31 from the University of Veterinary Sciences Brno, Czech Republic to Monika Dolejská.

References

Ahlstrom CA, Ramey AM, Woksepp H, Bonnedahl J (2019) Repeated Detection of Carbapenemase-Producing Escherichia coli in Gulls Inhabiting Alaska. Antimicrob Agents Chemother:63

Ahlstrom CA, Frick A, Pongratz C, Spink K, Xavier C, Bonnedahl J, Ramey AM (2021a) Genomic comparison of carbapenem-resistant Enterobacteriaceae from humans and gulls in Alaska. J Glob Antimicrob Resist 25:23–25

Ahlstrom CA, van Toor ML, Woksepp H et al (2021b) Evidence for continental-scale dispersal of antimicrobial resistant bacteria by landfill-foraging gulls. Sci Total Environ 764:144551

Ahlstrom CA, Scott LC, Woksepp H, Bonnedahl J, Ramey AM (2023a) Environmental antimicrobial resistance gene detection from wild bird habitats using two methods: a commercially available culture-independent qPCR assay and culture of indicator bacteria followed by whole-genome sequencing. J Glob Antimicrob Resist 33:186–193

Ahlstrom CA, Woksepp H, Sandegren L, Ramey AM, Bonnedahl J (2023b) Exchange of Carbapenem-resistant Escherichia coli sequence type 38 intercontinentally and among wild bird, human, and environmental niches. Appl Environ Microbiol 89:e0031923

Alam MU, Rahman M, Abdullah Al M, Islam MA, Asaduzzaman M, Sarker S, Rousham E, Unicomb L (2019) Human exposure to antimicrobial resistance from poultry production: assessing hygiene and waste-disposal practices in Bangladesh. Int J Hyg Environ Health 222:1068–1076

Allel K, Day L, Hamilton A, Lin L, Furuya-Kanamori L, Moore CE, Van Boeckel T, Laxminarayan R, Yakob L (2023) Global antimicrobial-resistance drivers: an ecological country-level study at the human-animal interface. Lancet Planet Health 7:e291–e303

Alvarez-Molina A, Cobo-Diaz JF, Alexa EA, Crispie F, Prieto M, Lopez M, Cotter PD, Alvarez-Ordonez A (2023) Sequencing-based analysis of the microbiomes of Spanish food processing facilities reveals environment-specific variation in the dominant taxa and antibiotic resistance genes. Food Res Int 173:113442

Anjum MF, Marco-Jimenez F, Duncan D, Marin C, Smith RP, Evans SJ (2019) Livestock-associated methicillin-resistant Staphylococcus aureus from animals and animal products in the UK. Front Microbiol 10:2136

Anjum MF, Schmitt H, Borjesson S, Berendonk TU & network W (2021) The potential of using E. coli as an indicator for the surveillance of antimicrobial resistance (AMR) in the environment. Curr Opin Microbiol 64: 152–158

Antimicrobial Resistance C (2022) Global burden of bacterial antimicrobial resistance in 2019: a systematic analysis. Lancet 399:629–655

Antunes P, Novais C, Peixe L (2020) Food-to-humans bacterial transmission. Microbiol Spectr 8

Araujo G, Yunta C, Terre M, Mereu A, Ipharraguerre I, Bach A (2015) Intestinal permeability and incidence of diarrhea in newborn calves. J Dairy Sci 98:7309–7317

Arthur TM, Brichta-Harhay DM, Bosilevac JM, Kalchayanand N, Shackelford SD, Wheeler TL, Koohmaraie M (2010) Super shedding of Escherichia coli O157:H7 by cattle and the impact on beef carcass contamination. Meat Sci 86:32–37

Atterby C, Borjesson S, Ny S, Jarhult JD, Byfors S, Bonnedahl J (2017) ESBL-producing Escherichia coli in Swedish gulls – a case of environmental pollution from humans? PLoS One 12:e0190380

Ben Yahia H, Chairat S, Gharsa H, Alonso CA, Ben Sallem R, Porres-Osante N, Hamdi N, Torres C, Ben Slama K (2020) First report of KPC-2 and KPC-3-producing enterobacteriaceae in wild birds in Africa. Microb Ecol 79:30–37

Bengtsson-Palme J, Kristiansson E, Larsson DGJ (2018) Environmental factors influencing the development and spread of antibiotic resistance. FEMS Microbiol Rev 42

Berdy J (2012) Thoughts and facts about antibiotics: where we are now and where we are heading. J Antibiot (Tokyo) 65:385–395

Betts JW, Hornsey M & La Ragione RM (2018) Novel antibacterials: alternatives to traditional antibiotics. Adv Microb Physiol 73: 123–169, Elsevier

Blaak H, Lynch G, Italiaander R, Hamidjaja RA, Schets FM, de Roda Husman AM (2015a) Multidrug-resistant and extended spectrum beta-lactamase-producing Escherichia coli in Dutch surface water and wastewater. PLoS One 10:e0127752

Blaak H, van Hoek AH, Hamidjaja RA, van der Plaats RQ, Kerkhof-de Heer L, de Roda Husman AM, Schets FM (2015b) Distribution, numbers, and diversity of ESBL-producing E. coli in the poultry farm environment. PloS One 10:e0135402

Blake LJ, Häsler B, Bennani H, Mateus AL, Eastmure E, Mays N, Stärk KD (2022) The UK antimicrobial resistance strategy 2013–18: a qualitative study of international and domestic policy and action related to livestock and the food chain. Front Sustain Food Systems 6

Bonnedahl J, Stedt J, Waldenstrom J, Svensson L, Drobni M, Olsen B (2015) Comparison of extended-spectrum beta-lactamase (ESBL) CTX-M genotypes in Franklin gulls from Canada and Chile. PLoS One 10:e0141315

Bos ME, Mevius DJ, Wagenaar JA, van Geijlswijk IM, Mouton JW, Heederik DJ, Netherlands Veterinary Medicines A (2015) Antimicrobial prescription patterns of veterinarians: introduction of a benchmarking approach. J Antimicrob Chemother 70:2423–2425

Bouma JE, Lenski RE (1988) Evolution of a bacteria/plasmid association. Nature 335:351–352

Broens EM, Graat EA, Van der Wolf PJ, Van de Giessen AW, De Jong MC (2011) Transmission of methicillin resistant Staphylococcus aureus among pigs during transportation from farm to abattoir. Vet J 189:302–305

Caekebeke N, Ringenier M, Jonquiere FJ et al (2021) Coaching Belgian and Dutch broiler farmers aimed at Antimicrobial stewardship and disease prevention. Antibiotics 10

Canadian IPfAR (2009) Salmonella Heidelberg Ceftiofur-related resistance in human and retail chicken isolates – 2006 to 2008. Canada Public Health Services. https://www.canada.ca/en/public-health/services/surveillance/canadian-integrated-program-antimicrobial-resistance-surveillance-cipars/update-salmonella-heidelberg-ceftiofur-related-resistance-human-retail-chicken-isolates-2006-2008.html

Cao J, Hu Y, Liu F, Wang Y, Bi Y, Lv N, Li J, Zhu B, Gao GF (2020) Metagenomic analysis reveals the microbiome and resistome in migratory birds. Microbiome 8:26

Chambers PG, Grandin T, Heinz G & Srisuva T (2001) Guidelines for humane handling, transport and slaughter of livestock Food and Agriculture Organization of the United Nations Regional Office for Asia and the Pacific

Chandrakar C, Shakya S, Patyal A, Jain A, Ali SL, Mishra OP (2022) ERIC-PCR-based molecular typing of multidrug-resistant Escherichia coli isolated from houseflies (Musca domestica) in the environment of milk and meat shops. Lett Appl Microbiol 75:1549–1558

Chmelikova E, Bolechova P, Chaloupkova H, Svobodova I, Jovicic M, Sedmikova M (2020) Salivary cortisol as a marker of acute stress in dogs: a review. Domest Anim Endocrinol 72:106428

Christaki E, Marcou M, Tofarides A (2020) Antimicrobial resistance in bacteria: mechanisms, evolution, and persistence. J Mol Evol 88:26–40

Cirone F, Padalino B, Tullio D, Capozza P, Lo Surdo M, Lanave G, Pratelli A (2019) Prevalence of pathogens related to bovine respiratory disease before and after transportation in beef steers: preliminary results. Animals (Basel), vol 9

Cobo-Angel C, Roche SM, LeBlanc SJ (2023) Understanding the role of veterinarians in antimicrobial stewardship on Canadian dairy farms: a mixed-methods study. PLoS One 18:e0289415

Collignon PJ, McEwen SA (2019) One health – its importance in helping to better control antimicrobial resistance. Trop Med Infect Dis 4

Cray WC Jr, Casey TA, Bosworth BT, Rasmussen MA (1998) Effect of dietary stress on fecal shedding of Escherichia coli O157:H7 in calves. Appl Environ Microbiol 64:1975–1979

Crescio MI, Mastrantonio G, Bertolini S et al (2021) Using network analysis to identify seasonal patterns and key nodes for risk-based surveillance of pig diseases in Italy. Transbound Emerg Dis 68:3541–3551

Dadgostar P (2019) Antimicrobial resistance: implications and costs. Infect Drug Resist 12:3903–3910

Davies R, Wales A (2019) Antimicrobial Resistance on farms: a review including biosecurity and the potential role of disinfectants in Resistance selection. Compr Rev Food Sci Food Saf 18:753–774

De Silva L, Wickramanayake M, Heo GJ (2021) Virulence and antimicrobial resistance potential of Aeromonas spp. associated with shellfish. Lett Appl Microbiol 73:176–186

Dewell GA, Simpson CA, Dewell RD et al (2008) Risk associated with transportation and lairage on hide contamination with Salmonella enterica in finished beef cattle at slaughter. J Food Prot 71:2228–2232

Djordjevic SP, Jarocki VM, Seemann T, Cummins ML, Watt AE, Drigo B, Wyrsch ER, Reid CJ, Donner E, Howden BP (2024) Genomic surveillance for antimicrobial resistance – a one health perspective. Nat Rev Genet 25:142–157

Dolejska M, Literak I (2019) Wildlife is overlooked in the epidemiology of medically important antibiotic-resistant bacteria. Antimicrob Agents Chemother 63

Dolejska M, Papagiannitsis CC (2018) Plasmid-mediated resistance is going wild. Plasmid 99:99–111

Duarte ASR, Stark KDC, Munk P et al (2020) Addressing learning needs on the use of metagenomics in antimicrobial resistance surveillance. Front Public Health 8:38
ECA ECoA (2023) Transports of live animals in the EU: challenges and opportunities
EFSA (2021) Role played by the environment in the emergence and spread of antimicrobial resistance (AMR) through the food chain. EFSA J 19:188
EMA EMA (2023) Sales of veterinary antimicrobial agents in 31 European countries in 2022. Luxembourg, p 94
Ferguson DM, Warner RD (2008) Have we underestimated the impact of pre-slaughter stress on meat quality in ruminants? Meat Sci 80:12–19
Fevre EM, Bronsvoort BM, Hamilton KA, Cleaveland S (2006) Animal movements and the spread of infectious diseases. Trends Microbiol 14:125–131
Fisher AD, Colditz IG, Lee C, Ferguson DM (2009) The influence of land transport on animal welfare in extensive farming systems. J Vet Behav 4:157–162
Franklin AB, Ramey AM, Bentler KT, Barrett NL, McCurdy LM, Ahlstrom CA, Bonnedahl J, Shriner SA, Chandler JC (2020) Gulls as sources of environmental contamination by Colistin-resistant bacteria. Sci Rep 10:4408
Frost I, Van Boeckel TP, Pires J, Craig J, Laxminarayan R (2019) Global geographic trends in antimicrobial resistance: the role of international travel. J Travel Med 26
Gay E, Bour M, Cazeau G, Jarrige N, Martineau C, Madec JY, Haenni M (2019) Antimicrobial usages and antimicrobial resistance in commensal Escherichia coli from veal calves in France: evolution during the fattening process. Front Microbiol 10:792
Giri S, Kudva V, Shetty K, Shetty V (2021) Prevalence and characterization of extended-spectrum beta-lactamase-producing antibiotic-resistant Escherichia coli and Klebsiella pneumoniae in ready-to-eat street foods. Antibiotics 10
Guardabassi L, Schwarz S, Lloyd DH (2004) Pet animals as reservoirs of antimicrobial-resistant bacteria. J Antimicrob Chemother 54:321–332
Guenther S, Wuttke J, Bethe A, Vojtech J, Schaufler K, Semmler T, Ulrich RG, Wieler LH, Ewers C (2013) Is fecal carriage of extended-spectrum-beta-lactamase-producing Escherichia coli in urban rats a risk for public health? Antimicrob Agents Chemother 57:2424–2425
Guenther S, Semmler T, Stubbe A, Stubbe M, Wieler LH, Schaufler K (2017) Chromosomally encoded ESBL genes in Escherichia coli of ST38 from Mongolian wild birds. J Antimicrob Chemother 72:1310–1313
Guiney DG, Fang FC, Krause M, Libby S, Buchmeier NA, Fierer J (1995) Biology and clinical significance of virulence plasmids in Salmonella serovars. Clin Infect Dis 21(Suppl 2):S146–S151
Haas CN (2020) Quantitative microbial risk assessment and molecular biology: paths to integration. Environ Sci Technol 54:8539–8546
Hansen TA, Joshi T, Larsen AR, Andersen PS, Harms K, Mollerup S, Willerslev E, Fuursted K, Nielsen LP, Hansen AJ (2016) Vancomycin gene selection in the microbiome of urban Rattus norvegicus from hospital environment. Evol Med Public Health 2016:219–226
Hasan B, Melhus A, Sandegren L, Alam M, Olsen B (2014) The gull (Chroicocephalus brunnicephalus) as an environmental bioindicator and reservoir for antibiotic resistance on the coastlines of the Bay of Bengal. Microb Drug Resist 20:466–471
Hassena AB, Belmabrouk S, Amor MG, Zormati S, Guermazi-Toumi S, Siala-Trigui M, Gdoura R (2022) Study of virulence genes, antimicrobial resistance, and genetic relatedness of foodborne salmonella isolates from Tunisia. J Food Prot 85:1779–1789
Jamborova I, Johnston BD, Papousek I et al (2018) Extensive genetic commonality among wildlife, wastewater, community, and nosocomial isolates of Escherichia coli sequence type 131 (H30R1 and H30Rx subclones) that carry bla(CTX-M-27) or bla(CTX-M-15). Antimicrob Agents Chemother 62
Jarrige N, Cazeau G, Morignat E, Chanteperdrix M, Gay E (2017) Quantitative and qualitative analysis of antimicrobial usage in white veal calves in France. Prev Vet Med 144:158–166
Jin L, Li J, Nation RL, Nicolazzo JA (2012) Effect of systemic infection induced by Pseudomonas aeruginosa on the brain uptake of colistin in mice. Antimicrob Agents Chemother 56:5240–5246

Joat NN, Khan S, Chousalkar K (2021) Understanding the effects of intramuscular injection and feed withdrawal on Salmonella typhimurium shedding and gut microbiota in pullets. J Anim Sci Biotechnol 12:78

Koorakula R, Schiavinato M, Ghanbari M, Wegl G, Grabner N, Koestelbauer A, Klose V, Dohm JC, Domig KJ (2022) Metatranscriptomic analysis of the chicken gut resistome response to in-feed antibiotics and natural feed additives. Front Microbiol 13:833790

Kozak GK, Boerlin P, Janecko N, Reid-Smith RJ, Jardine C (2009) Antimicrobial resistance in Escherichia coli isolates from swine and wild small mammals in the proximity of swine farms and in natural environments in Ontario, Canada. Appl Environ Microbiol 75:559–566

Lambraki IA, Cousins M, Graells T et al (2022) Factors influencing antimicrobial resistance in the European food system and potential leverage points for intervention: a participatory, One Health study. PloS One 17:e0263914

Larsson DGJ, Flach CF (2022) Antibiotic resistance in the environment. Nat Rev Microbiol 20:257–269

Leger A, Lambraki I, Graells T et al (2021) AMR-intervene: a social-ecological framework to capture the diversity of actions to tackle antimicrobial resistance from a One Health perspective. J Antimicrob Chemother 76:1–21

Liguori K, Keenum I, Davis BC, Calarco J, Milligan E, Harwood VJ, Pruden A (2022) Antimicrobial resistance monitoring of water environments: a framework for standardized methods and quality control. Environ Sci Technol 56:9149–9160

Lima LM, Silva B, Barbosa G, Barreiro EJ (2020a) Beta-lactam antibiotics: an overview from a medicinal chemistry perspective. Eur J Med Chem 208:112829

Lima T, Domingues S, Da Silva GJ (2020b) Manure as a potential hotspot for antibiotic resistance dissemination by horizontal gene transfer events. Vet Sci 7

Lin Y, Zhang L, Wu J, Yang K (2023) Wild birds-the sentinel of antibiotic resistance for urban river: study on egrets and Jinjiang river in Chengdu, China. Environ Res 216:114566

Llewelyn MJ, Fitzpatrick JM, Darwin E, SarahTonkin C, Gorton C, Paul J, Peto TEA, Yardley L, Hopkins S, Walker AS (2017) The antibiotic course has had its day. BMJ 358:j3418

Loncaric I, Stalder GL, Mehinagic K, Rosengarten R, Hoelzl F, Knauer F, Walzer C (2013) Comparison of ESBL – and AmpC producing Enterobacteriaceae and methicillin-resistant Staphylococcus aureus (MRSA) isolated from migratory and resident population of rooks (Corvus frugilegus) in Austria. PLoS One 8:e84048

Loucif L, Chelaghma W, Bendjama E, Cherak Z, Khellaf M, Khemri A, Rolain JM (2022) Detection of bla(OXA-48) and mcr-1 genes in Escherichia coli isolates from pigeon (Columba livia) in Algeria. Microorganisms 10

Lunha K, Leangapichart T, Jiwakanon J, Angkititrakul S, Sunde M, Jarhult JD, Strom Hallenberg G, Hickman RA, Van Boeckel T & Magnusson U (2020) Antimicrobial Resistance in fecal Escherichia coli from humans and pigs at farms at different levels of intensification. Antibiotics 9

Magistrali C, Dionisi AM, De Curtis P, Cucco L, Vischi O, Scuota S, Zicavo A, Pezzotti G (2008) Contamination of Salmonella spp. in a pig finishing herd, from the arrival of the animals to the slaughterhouse. Res Vet Sci 85:204–207

Manaia CM (2017) Assessing the risk of antibiotic resistance transmission from the environment to humans: non-direct proportionality between abundance and risk. Trends Microbiol 25:173–181

Mannion C, Egan J, Lynch BP, Fanning S, Leonard N (2008) An investigation into the efficacy of washing trucks following the transportation of pigs – a salmonella perspective. Foodborne Pathog Dis 5:261–271

Marcelino VR, Wille M, Hurt AC et al (2019) Meta-transcriptomics reveals a diverse antibiotic resistance gene pool in avian microbiomes. BMC Biol 17:31

Martin-Pelaez S, Peralta B, Creus E, Dalmau A, Velarde A, Perez JF, Mateu E, Martin-Orue SM (2009) Different feed withdrawal times before slaughter influence caecal fermentation and faecal Salmonella shedding in pigs. Vet J 182:469–473

Martin-Velez V, Navarro J, Figuerola J, Aymi R, Sabate S, Planell R, Vila J, Montalvo T (2024) A spatial analysis of urban gulls contribution to the potential spread of zoonotic and antibiotic-resistant bacteria. Sci Total Environ 912:168762

Massacci FR, Morelli A, Cucco L, Castinel A, Ortenzi R, Tofani S, Pezzotti G, Estelle J, Paniccia M, Magistrali CF (2020) Transport to the slaughterhouse affects the salmonella shedding and modifies the fecal microbiota of finishing pigs. Animals (Basel) 10

Mathys DA, Mathys BA, Mollenkopf DF, Daniels JB, Wittum TE (2017) Enterobacteriaceae harboring AmpC (bla(CMY)) and ESBL (bla(CTX-M)) in migratory and nonmigratory wild songbird populations on Ohio Dairies. Vector Borne Zoonotic Dis 17:254–259

McEwen SA, Collignon PJ (2018) Antimicrobial Resistance: a One Health Perspective. Microbiol Spectr 6

McInnes RS, McCallum GE, Lamberte LE, van Schaik W (2020) Horizontal transfer of antibiotic resistance genes in the human gut microbiome. Curr Opin Microbiol 53:35–43

McIver KS, Amoako DG, Abia ALK, Bester LA, Chenia HY, Essack SY (2020) Molecular epidemiology of antibiotic-resistant Escherichia coli from farm-to-fork in intensive poultry production in KwaZulu-Natal, South Africa. Antibiotics 9

McMullin P (2022) Infectious diseases in free-range compared to conventional poultry production. Avian Pathol 51:424–434

Meyer E, Gastmeier P, Kola A, Schwab F (2012) Pet animals and foreign travel are risk factors for colonisation with extended-spectrum beta-lactamase-producing Escherichia coli. Infection 40:685–687

Miranda-de la Lama GC, Villarroel M, Maria GA (2014) Livestock transport from the perspective of the pre-slaughter logistic chain: a review. Meat Sci 98:9–20

Molechan C, Amoako DG, Abia ALK, Somboro AM, Bester LA, Essack SY (2019) Molecular epidemiology of antibiotic-resistant enterococcus spp. from the farm-to-fork continuum in intensive poultry production in KwaZulu-Natal, South Africa. Sci Total Environ 692:868–878

Mughini-Gras L, Dorado-Garcia A, van Duijkeren E et al (2019) Attributable sources of community-acquired carriage of Escherichia coli containing beta-lactam antibiotic resistance genes: a population-based modelling study. Lancet Planet Health 3:e357–e369

Mulchandani R, Wang Y, Gilbert M, Van Boeckel TP (2023) Global trends in antimicrobial use in food-producing animals: 2020 to 2030. PLOS Glob Public Health 3:e0001305

Münch B, Wochenschr T, Seedorf J, Schmidt R-G (2017) Open access animal transport vehicles as potential bioaerosol emitters: a preliminary contribution to environmental hygiene by means of computational fluid dynamics (CFD) simulation Tiertransportfahrzeuge als potenzielle Bioaerosol-Emittenten: Ein vorläufiger Beitrag zur Umwelthygiene unter Verwendung einer numerischen Strömungssimulation. Tierärztliche Wochenschrift 130:288–292

Nelson M, Jones SH, Edwards C, Ellis JC (2008) Characterization of Escherichia coli populations from gulls, landfill trash, and wastewater using ribotyping. Dis Aquat Org 81:53–63

Nesporova K, Wyrsch ER, Valcek A, Bitar I, Chaw K, Harris P, Hrabak J, Literak I, Djordjevic SP, Dolejska M (2020) Escherichia coli sequence type 457 is an emerging extended-spectrum-beta-lactam-resistant lineage with reservoirs in wildlife and food-producing animals. Antimicrob Agents Chemother 65

Nesporova K, Ruzickova M, Tarabai H, Krejci S, Masarikova M, Lausova J, Literak I, Dolejska M (2024) Changing dynamics of antibiotic resistant Escherichia in Caspian gulls shows the importance of longitudinal environmental studies. Environ Int 186:108606

Nguyen XD, Zhao Y, Evans JD, Lin J, Purswell JL (2022) Survival of Escherichia coli in airborne and settled poultry litter particles. Animals (Basel) 12

Nicolaisen S, Langkabel N, Thoene-Reineke C, Wiegard M (2023) Animal welfare during transport and slaughter of cattle: a systematic review of studies in the European legal framework. Animals (Basel) 13

Nielsen BL, Dybkjaer L, Herskin MS (2011) Road transport of farm animals: effects of journey duration on animal welfare. Animal 5:415–427

Novais C, Freitas AR, Silveira E, Antunes P, Silva R, Coque TM, Peixe L (2013) Spread of multidrug-resistant enterococcus to animals and humans: an underestimated role for the pig farm environment. J Antimicrob Chemother 68:2746–2754
OIE WOfAH (2015) OIE list of antimicrobial agents of veterinary importance. OIE, Paris
Padalino B, Raidal SL (2020) Effects of transport conditions on behavioural and physiological responses of horses. Animals (Basel) 10
Padalino B, Raidal SL, Hall E, Knight P, Celi P, Jeffcott L, Muscatello G (2016) A survey on transport management practices associated with injuries and health problems in horses. PLoS One 11:e0162371
Padalino B, Barrasso R, Tullio D, Zappaterra M, Costa LN, Bozzo G (2020) Protection of animals during transport: analysis of the infringements reported from 2009 to 2013 during on-road inspections in Italy. Animals (Basel) 10
Partridge SR, Kwong SM, Firth N, Jensen SO (2018) Mobile genetic elements associated with antimicrobial resistance. Clin Microbiol Rev 31
Patil A, Banerji R, Kanojiya P, Saroj SD (2021) Foodborne ESKAPE biofilms and antimicrobial resistance: lessons learned from clinical isolates. Pathog Glob Health 115:339–356
Picot V, Rasuli A, Abella-Rider A et al (2017) The Middle East and Eastern Europe rabies expert bureau (MEEREB) third meeting: Lyon-France (7–8 April, 2015). J Infect Public Health 10:695–701
Pires SM, Duarte AS, Hald T (2018) Source attribution and risk assessment of antimicrobial resistance. Microbiol Spectr 6
Pisoni L, Devant M, Blanch M, Pastor JJ, Marti S (2022) Simulation of feed restriction and fasting: effects on animal recovery and gastrointestinal permeability in unweaned Angus-Holstein calves. J Dairy Sci 105:2572–2586
Plaza PI, Lambertucci SA (2017) How are garbage dumps impacting vertebrate demography, health, and conservation? Global Ecol Conserv 12:9–20
Pratelli A, Cirone F, Capozza P, Trotta A, Corrente M, Balestrieri A, Buonavoglia C (2021) Bovine respiratory disease in beef calves supported long transport stress: an epidemiological study and strategies for control and prevention. Res Vet Sci 135:450–455
Pulingam T, Parumasivam T, Gazzali AM, Sulaiman AM, Chee JY, Lakshmanan M, Chin CF, Sudesh K (2022) Antimicrobial resistance: prevalence, economic burden, mechanisms of resistance and strategies to overcome. Eur J Pharm Sci 170:106103
Qian M, Xu D, Wang J, Zaeim D, Han J, Qu D (2023) Isolation, antimicrobial resistance and virulence characterization of Salmonella spp. from fresh foods in retail markets in Hangzhou, China. PLoS One 18:e0292621
Ramey AM, Ahlstrom CA (2020) Antibiotic resistant bacteria in wildlife: perspectives on trends, acquisition and dissemination, data gaps, and future directions. J Wildl Dis 56:1–15
Rule AM, Evans SL, Silbergeld EK (2008) Food animal transport: a potential source of community exposures to health hazards from industrial farming (CAFOs). J Infect Public Health 1:33–39
Sandegren L, Stedt J, Lustig U, Bonnedahl J, Andersson DI, Jarhult JD (2018) Long-term carriage and rapid transmission of extended spectrum beta-lactamase-producing E. coli within a flock of Mallards in the absence of antibiotic selection. Environ Microbiol Rep 10:576–582
Savin M, Bierbaum G, Hammerl JA, Heinemann C, Parcina M, Sib E, Voigt A, Kreyenschmidt J (2020) ESKAPE bacteria and extended-spectrum-beta-lactamase-producing Escherichia coli isolated from wastewater and process water from German poultry slaughterhouses. Appl Environ Microbiol 86
Schmithausen R, Schulze-Geisthoevel S, Heinemann C, Bierbaum G, Exner M, Petersen B, Steinhoff-Wagner J (2018) Reservoirs and transmission pathways of resistant indicator bacteria in the biotope pig stable and along the food chain: a review from a one health perspective. Sustainability 10
Schwartzkopf-Genswein KS, Faucitano L, Dadgar S, Shand P, Gonzalez LA, Crowe TG (2012) Road transport of cattle, swine and poultry in North America and its impact on animal welfare, carcass and meat quality: a review. Meat Sci 92:227–243

Scott HM, Acuff G, Bergeron G et al (2019) Critically important antibiotics: criteria and approaches for measuring and reducing their use in food animal agriculture. Ann N Y Acad Sci 1441:8–16
Sharma L, Nagpal R, Jackson CR, Patel D, Singh P (2021) Antibiotic-resistant bacteria and gut microbiome communities associated with wild-caught shrimp from the United States versus imported farm-raised retail shrimp. Sci Rep 11:3356
Simoes RR, Poirel L, Da Costa PM, Nordmann P (2010) Seagulls and beaches as reservoirs for multidrug-resistant Escherichia coli. Emerg Infect Dis 16:110–112
Sora VM, Meroni G, Martino PA, Soggiu A, Bonizzi L, Zecconi A (2021) Extraintestinal pathogenic Escherichia coli: virulence factors and antibiotic resistance. Pathogens 10
Sterchi M, Faverjon C, Sarasua C, Vargas ME, Berezowski J, Bernstein A, Grutter R, Nathues H (2019) The pig transport network in Switzerland: structure, patterns, and implications for the transmission of infectious diseases between animal holdings. PLoS One 14:e0217974
Swift BMC, Bennett M, Waller K et al (2019) Anthropogenic environmental drivers of antimicrobial resistance in wildlife. Sci Total Environ 649:12–20
Tateo A, Nanni Costa L, Padalino B (2022) The welfare of dogs and cats during transport in Europe: a literature review. Ital J Anim Sci 21:539–550
Tenhagen BA, Alt K, Pfefferkorn B, Wiehle L, Kasbohrer A, Fetsch A (2018) Short communication: methicillin-resistant Staphylococcus aureus in conventional and organic dairy herds in Germany. J Dairy Sci 101:3380–3386
Ter Kuile BH, Kraupner N, Brul S (2016) The risk of low concentrations of antibiotics in agriculture for resistance in human health care. FEMS Microbiol Lett 363
Titouche Y, Akkou M, Houali K, Auvray F, Hennekinne JA (2022) Role of milk and milk products in the spread of methicillin-resistant Staphylococcus aureus in the dairy production chain. J Food Sci 87:3699–3723
Tsiouris V, Georgopoulou I, Batzios C, Pappaioannou N, Ducatelle R, Fortomaris P (2014) Temporary feed restriction partially protects broilers from necrotic enteritis. Avian Pathol 43:139–145
Valadez-Noriega M, Estevez-Moreno LX, Rayas-Amor AA, Rubio-Lozano MS, Galindo F, Miranda-de la Lama GC (2018) Livestock hauliers' attitudes, knowledge and current practices towards animal welfare, occupational wellbeing and transport risk factors: a Mexican survey. Prev Vet Med 160:76–84
Valkova L, Vecerek V, Voslarova E, Kaluza M, Takacova D, Brscic M (2022) Animal welfare during transport: comparison of mortality during transport from farm to slaughter of different animal species and categories in The Czech Republic. Ital J Anim Sci 21:914–923
Veldman KT, Wit B, Franz E, Heederik DJJ (2023) Monitoring of antimicrobial resistance and antibiotic usage in animals in The Netherlands in 2022. Wageningen Bioveterinary Research (WBVR), Lelystad, p 76
Verbrugghe E, Boyen F, Van Parys A, Van Deun K, Croubels S, Thompson A, Shearer N, Leyman B, Haesebrouck F, Pasmans F (2011) Stress induced salmonella Typhimurium recrudescence in pigs coincides with cortisol induced increased intracellular proliferation in macrophages. Vet Res 42:118
Vikesland P, Garner E, Gupta S, Kang S, Maile-Moskowitz A, Zhu N (2019) Differential drivers of antimicrobial resistance across the world. Acc Chem Res 52:916–924
von Tippelskirch P, Golz G, Projahn M, Daehre K, Friese A, Roesler U, Alter T, Orquera S (2018) Prevalence and quantitative analysis of ESBL and AmpC beta-lactamase producing Enterobacteriaceae in broiler chicken during slaughter in Germany. Int J Food Microbiol 281:82–89
WHO (2016) Critically important antimicrobials for human medicine, 4th revision. WHO, Geneva
Wink PL, Lima-Morales D, Meurer R, Barth AL (2022) Escherichia coli carrying Bla(NDM-1) obtained from a migratory penguin (Spheniscus magellanicus) in the Brazilian seacoast. Braz J Microbiol 53:499–502
WOAH WOoAH (2023a) Aquatic animal health code
WOAH WOoAH (2023b) Terrestial animal health code

Wyrsch ER, Nesporova K, Tarabai H, Jamborova I, Bitar I, Literak I, Dolejska M, Djordjevic SP (2022) Urban wildlife crisis: Australian Silver Gull is a bystander host to widespread clinical antibiotic resistance. mSystems 7:e0015822

Zeng H, De Reu K, Gabriel S, Mattheus W, De Zutter L, Rasschaert G (2021) Salmonella prevalence and persistence in industrialized poultry slaughterhouses. Poult Sci 100:100991

Zhao J, Jin L, Wu D et al (2022) Global airborne bacterial community-interactions with Earth's microbiomes and anthropogenic activities. Proc Natl Acad Sci USA 119:e2204465119

Zinsstag J, Kaiser-Grolimund A, Heitz-Tokpa K et al (2023) Advancing one human-animal-environment health for global health security: what does the evidence say? Lancet 401:591–604

Chapter 5
Fluoroquinolones: Role in Healthcare and Environmental Impact and Resistance Development

Lisa Teichmann

Abstract Fluoroquinolones are highly effective antimicrobials for treating a variety of infections. There are four generations that differ in chemical structure. The pater generations are more effective than the earlier ones. Fluoroquinolones inhibit DNA replication by inhibiting bacterial DNA gyrase and topoisomerase IV. Resistance rapidly arises due to mutations in these enzymes. Other enzymes can protect the target enzymes from inhibition by fluoroquinolones. In addition, the SOS-response can lead to rapid development of resistance. A more detailed understanding of the mode of action and the processes causing the build-up of resistance is needed to prevent unnecessary resistance as a result of treatment with this class of antimicrobials.

Keywords Fluoroquinolones · Multidrug-resistant infections · Veterinary medicine · Transfer of resistance

Introduction

Fluoroquinolones (FQs) are broad-spectrum antibiotics that play a vital role in modern medicine, effectively treating a wide range of bacterial infections. Their efficacy against Gram-positive and Gram-negative bacteria, including common pathogens such as *Escherichia coli*, *Staphylococcus aureus*, and *Pseudomonas aeruginosa*, makes them indispensable (Hooper 1998). Despite growing concerns over potential severe side effects (EMA 2023), FQs remain a cornerstone in the treatment of multidrug-resistant (MDR) infections, including MDR tuberculosis, offering a critical option when other antibiotics fail (World Health Organization 2019).

L. Teichmann (✉)
Department of Molecular Biology and Microbial Food Safety, Swammerdam Institute of Life Sciences, University of Amsterdam, Amsterdam, The Netherlands
e-mail: lisa@teichmann-sdw.de

B. ter Kuile (ed.), *Antimicrobial Resistance and Antibiotics Usage in Livestock*,
https://doi.org/10.1007/978-3-032-04598-0_5

Since their introduction in the 1980s, FQs have seen widespread use in clinical settings, with their application extending to veterinary medicine in the 1990s (Bhatt and Chatterjee 2022). However, resistance soon followed. By the mid-1990s, clinical isolates of *Staphylococcus aureus* and *Pseudomonas aeruginosa* exhibiting reduced susceptibility to FQs were reported (File Jr. 1999; Dalhoff 2012). As FQ use escalated, so did the incidence of resistance. By the late 1990s and early 2000s, resistance was no longer confined to hospital-acquired infections but had also spread to the community (Goossens and Sprenger 1998). This universal use, across both human and veterinary medicine, has further aggravated environmental contamination, positioning FQs as significant ecological pollutants (Bhatt and Chatterjee 2022).

Bacteria exposed to sub-lethal concentrations of FQs can acquire resistance through genetic mutations or the horizontal transfer of ARGs (Rusu et al. 2015). This compromises the efficacy of FQs and contributes to the broader issue of antibiotic resistance in the environment. Fluoroquinolones (FQs) are known for their chemical stability, enabling them to persist in the environment for extended periods (Van Doorslaer et al. 2014). Their resistance to degradation processes, such as photolysis and biodegradation, allows them to remain active and potentially bioavailable long after their initial use (Van Doorslaer et al. 2014). This environmental persistence is further exacerbated by their ability to adsorb onto soil particles, leading to prolonged contamination of terrestrial ecosystems (Rosendahl et al. 2012). The presence of FQs in the environment exerts significant selective pressure on microbial communities, fostering the development and spread of antibiotic resistance genes (ARGs).

Over time, FQs have been studied using various methodological approaches, causing differences in the measurement of mutation rates or the definition of resistance thresholds, thereby complicating the interpretation and comparison of results across studies.

This paper aims to identify areas of disagreement and methodological inconsistencies in fluoroquinolone research in order to provide a clearer framework for future investigations. On the basis of such research, it should be possible to better inform both clinical users and improve the environmental management of FQs.

Implications of the Chemical Structure

Fluoroquinolones (FQs) are a subclass of the synthetic quinolone antibiotics that were developed in the 1980s by introducing a fluorine atom at the C-6 position of the quinolone core structure (Naeem et al. 2016). This structural modification significantly expanded their antibacterial spectrum, improved potency, and enhanced pharmacokinetic properties (reviewed in (Pham et al. 2019)). Additionally, modifying substituents at specific positions further enhanced the drugs' lipophilicity, allowing better cell penetration and improved half-life (Brighty and Gootz 1997, 2000; Ball 2000; Domagala 1994).

These chemical advancements led to the development of several generations of fluoroquinolones, each offering improved efficacy and broader antimicrobial activity:

- **First Generation**: Includes drugs like norfloxacin, with enhanced activity against Gram-negative bacteria but limited effectiveness against Gram-positive organisms.
- **Second Generation**: Contains ciprofloxacin and enrofloxacin, with a broader activity that encompasses both Gram-negative and some Gram-positive bacteria.
- **Third Generation**: Includes levofloxacin, which offers improved activity against Gram-positive bacteria while retaining efficacy against Gram-negative organisms.
- **Fourth Generation**: Contains moxifloxacin, which has enhanced activity against anaerobic bacteria and improved efficacy against resistant Gram-positive organisms.

The differences in properties such as hydrophobicity due to the distinct chemical structures of each FQ not only influence their ability to penetrate bacterial cells and reach their cellular targets but also impact the resistance mechanisms that bacteria develop and are therefore important to consider for FQ resistance research (Piddock et al. 2001; Denis and Moreau 1993). For example, moxifloxacin, with its complex molecular structure, is less likely to be targeted by efflux pumps as the primary resistance mechanism (Pestova et al. 2000). Similarly, sparfloxacin's high hydrophobicity also reduces its susceptibility to efflux-mediated excretion (Zhanel et al. 1999).

Pharmacokinetics and -Dynamics

Many pharmacodynamic doctrines for fluoroquinolones (FQs) have been deduced from those established for aminoglycosides, another concentration-dependent antibiotic class (Wright et al. 2000). In contrast to time-dependent drugs, where efficacy pivots on how long the drug concentration remains above the MIC (minimum inhibitory concentration), concentration-dependent agents exert greater antimicrobial activity as their concentration increases. For these drugs, the rate and extent of bacterial killing correlate with peak drug levels or the overall drug exposure over time. While the pharmacokinetic profiles of some FQ agents have been reviewed (Wright et al. 2000; Aminimanizani et al. 2001), optimal dosing regimens for FQs across different pathogens or disease states have yet to be established. One challenge lies in the inconsistency of methodologies, particularly in *in vitro* studies. Currently, there seems to be no consensus on key experimental factors such as log reduction endpoints, experiment duration, inoculum size, regrowth, and how to prevent antibiotic carryover (Wright et al. 2000). Furthermore, differences in MIC testing methods—whether Etest, broth microdilution, or disc diffusion—introduce variability into the data, complicating comparisons across studies. Environmental factors, such as the infection site and pH variations, can also affect MIC results, underscoring the critical need for standardized research protocols to achieve more reliable and reproducible data.

Mode of Action

While it is generally known that FQs inhibit bacterial DNA gyrase and topoisomerase IV, essential enzymes for DNA replication and repair (Hooper 1999, 2001)—the specific interactions and differential impacts of individual FQ on these targets are not fully understood and remain subjects of ongoing research and debate (Madurga et al. 2008; Ojkic et al. 2020). FQs exert their bactericidal action by stabilizing the enzyme-DNA complexes that form during the catalytic cycles of DNA gyrase and topoisomerase IV, ultimately inducing lethal double-stranded DNA breaks (Bush et al. 2020). Recent research suggests that there is a FQ-specific ability to stabilize this gyrase-DNA-cleaved complex, which not only plays a role in the formation of persister cells but also influences the cleavage strength and location within the enzyme (Tang and Brynildsen 2023). This distinct stabilization mechanism may help explain the varying resistance profiles associated with different FQs, as it is likely to influence the ability of each FQ to inhibit DNA supercoiling and relaxation and thus exploit their bactericidal activity based on the DNA gyrase target.

The chemical structure of each FQ plays a crucial role in determining its binding affinity and specificity for these enzymes (Madurga et al. 2008; Higgins et al. 2003). Even minor structural differences among FQ compounds can significantly influence how they interact with DNA gyrase and topoisomerase IV, impacting not only their efficacy but also their role in resistance development. While both enzymes are targeted by FQs, individual drugs may exhibit a preference for one over the other, contributing to variability in their antibacterial effectiveness (Fournier et al. 2000). Resistance to FQs typically arises through mutations in the genes encoding DNA gyrase or topoisomerase IV, which modify drug binding sites and decrease susceptibility (Bryskier 1993; Teichmann et al. 2025). The nature and frequency of these mutations vary with the specific FQ used, leading to distinct resistance profiles within the same species (Teichmann et al. 2025).

Unknown Lethality Mechanisms

FQ kill bacteria in a concentration-dependent manner (Wright et al. 2000). The process begins with the binding of the drug to a topoisomerase-DNA cleavage complex. What happens next—whether the cell dies swiftly or lingers—depends not only on the FQ concentration but also on whether this complex is further processed. This processing involves the conversion of the stabilized cleavage complex into irreversible double-strand breaks, a lethal event that ultimately seals the cell's fate (Bush et al. 2020).

During slow death, the replication forks and transcription bubbles are arrested and thus DNA and RNA synthesis is halted (Bush et al. 2020). Because this inhibition is reversible and thus unlikely to cause cell death, the exact cause of lethality occurring during long FQ treatments at low concentrations remains unclear. In contrast, rapid death occurs at high FQ concentrations in a protein-synthesis-dependent or -independent manner. It appears when the quinolone-poisoned gyrase subunits dissociate or are removed from the DNA (Bush et al. 2020). In the protein-synthesis-dependent pathway, lethality is thought to result from proteins that remove gyrase from the DNA, leading to the release of double-stranded DNA breaks and subsequent cell death (Bush et al. 2020). However, the identity of the proteins involved in this process remains unknown. In the protein-synthesis-independent pathway, lethality likely occurs due to the dissociation of gyrase subunits, which also results in the release of fatal double-strand breaks (Chen et al. 1996).

Drug-Specific Resistance Profiles

Historically, based on genetic studies in *E. coli* and *Streptococcus pneumoniae*, it was believed that DNA gyrase served as the primary target in Gram-negative bacteria and topoisomerase IV in Gram-positive strains (Khodursky et al. 1995; Aedo and Tse-Dinh 2012; Pan et al. 1996). While this has been disproven by now for different quinolones and species (Pan and Fisher 1997, 1998), there is still a knowledge gap about the species- and drug-specific targets of FQ. In *Streptococcus pneumoniae*, for instance, the primary target varies depending on the specific fluoroquinolone used. For example, ciprofloxacin, levofloxacin, moxifloxacin, and trovafloxacin primarily target the *parC* gene, while gatifloxacin and sparfloxacin target *gyrA* as their primary mechanism (Fukuda and Hiramatsu 1999). Computational binding studies indicate that CIP and LEV show very similar binding affinities to the DNA gyrase GyrA, whereas MOX shows unique binding patterns (Madurga et al. 2008). This variability in binding affinities may lead to unique resistance patterns, as mutations that affect binding can have different impacts depending on the specific FQ. Some mutations may still allow the drug to stabilize the DNA cleavage complex, while others may render the antibiotic ineffective.

Bacterial DNA gyrases share significant amino acid homology, particularly in the quinolone resistance determining region (QRDR), which spans amino acids 70–141 (Higgins et al. 2003). However, despite this homology, clear distinctions exist between Gram-positive and Gram-negative bacteria in this region. Even within the Gram-negative group, where the QRDRs are nearly identical, the DNA gyrases exhibit varying affinities for fluoroquinolones (Higgins et al. 2003). These differences in binding affinities influence species-specific susceptibility to FQs, contributing to the variability in resistance development. Topoisomerase IV, in contrast, shows less homology between species, with more pronounced differences between Gram-positive and Gram-negative bacteria. It however remains unclear whether these variations contribute to the distinctions between primary and secondary targets of fluoroquinolones (Higgins et al. 2003).

Next to mutations in the cellular targets, so-called qnr proteins are known to protect bacterial DNA gyrase and topoisomerase IV from the inhibitory effects of fluoroquinolones, thereby contributing to resistance (Tran et al. 2005; Jacoby et al.

2015). The expression of qnr genes, which contribute to quinolone resistance, can vary depending on the specific fluoroquinolone antibiotic used. The relative expression of qnr genes is differentially induced by various fluoroquinolones, such as CIP, LEV, and MOX (Briales et al. 2012). This differential induction suggests that the interaction between the antibiotic and the bacterial cell can influence the degree of resistance gene expression. Interestingly, the expression of qnr genes has also been linked to the induction of the SOS response (Briales et al. 2012; Da Re et al. 2009), suggesting that each FQ induces the SOS response to a different extend. It has been described that MOX induces the SOS response to a lesser extent than CIP, while reducing the growth rate less (Vestergaard et al. 2015).

Mutation Rate Measurements

Mutation rate measurements following fluoroquinolone exposure show significant variability across studies, often due to differences in experimental conditions, genetic backgrounds, and methodological approaches. These inconsistencies make it challenging to draw definitive conclusions about FQs mutation-inducing potential. For example, commonly used methods for measuring mutation rates, such as fluctuation assays and whole-genome sequencing, can yield varying results depending on the specific approach and parameters employed (Williams 2014). Additionally, variations in antibiotic concentrations—ranging from sub-lethal to minimum inhibitory concentration (MIC) levels and higher—complicate direct comparisons between studies. The SOS response, which plays a key role in driving mutation rates, is generally most strongly induced at sub-MIC levels (Torres-Barceló et al. 2015). However, factors such as nutrient availability and bacterial growth rate also modulate the extent of SOS activation, further complicating the interpretation of experimental outcomes (Jaramillo-Riveri et al. 2022).

The Role of the SOS Response

The cellular response to FQ-induced DNA damage involves complex regulatory pathways, which can modulate the bactericidal activity of FQs (Drlica et al. 2008). The extent to which different FQs activate these pathways and the resulting cellular outcomes can vary, contributing to differences in their antibacterial properties. One area of interest is the role of the SOS response, a bacterial defence mechanism activated by DNA damage, in mediating the effects of different fluoroquinolones (Da Re et al. 2009; Beaber et al. 2004). The SOS response, regulated by the RecA protein and the LexA repressor, arranges the expression of numerous genes involved in DNA repair and mutagenesis (Walker 1996; Janion 2008; Maslowska et al. 2019). Therefore, disrupting the RecA protein, which is pivotal in initiating the SOS response, has been a common experimental approach to studying the impacts of impairing this pathway (Diaz-Diaz et al. 2021; Recacha et al. 2017; Mo et al. 2016;

Urios et al. 1991; Singh et al. 2010; Alam et al. 2016; Da Silva Ribeiro et al. 2020; Bunnell et al. 2017; Thi et al. 2011). Another common method for investigating the effect of a disrupted SOS response is using strains that unable to cleave LexA, thereby preventing the transcription of the SOS operon (Cirz et al. 2005; Selwood et al. 2018; Maso et al. 2022). These models, while both affecting the SOS response pathway, have distinct biological impacts.

While the complete loss of RecA impacts homologous recombination and DNA repair, strains with an impaired LexA-cleavage still possess a functional recombination process. Comparisons between these methods should be carefully studied when interpreting experimental results. For instance, the total absence of RecA could result in a higher sensitivity to DNA damage beyond the scope of FQ action, affecting the overall bacterial survival and fitness. Knocking out recA indeed has a bigger impact on susceptibility to FQ than an impaired LexA cleavage (Recacha et al. 2017). Conversely, strains that cannot cleave LexA may specifically highlight the role of the SOS response in FQ-induced stress without broadly compromising other repair mechanisms. Indeed, it has been reported that a recA knockout showed reduced fitness in comparison to the wild-type strain (Recacha et al. 2019). Furthermore, the impact of knocking out recA on resistance development differs between species (Recacha et al. 2019). This difference may be attributed to varying reduced mutation rates in recA knockout mutants (Recacha et al. 2019), which might depend on the species.

In *Pseudomonas aeruginosa,* LexA mutants have reduced mutation rates in comparison to the respective wild-type; however, the observed reduced fitness did not influence evolvability when exposed to sub-lethal antibiotic regimes (Torres-Barceló et al. 2015). On the contrary, the strains adapted more rapidly to ciprofloxacin when LexA was impaired (Torres-Barceló et al. 2015). It must be noted that mutation rates vary strongly between fluoroquinolones, and different adaptive mutations lead to substantial variations in fitness and mutation rates depending on the antibiotic (Vestergaard et al. 2015; Schedletzky et al. 1999). Moreover, we still do not fully understand the SOS response and the multitude of proteins involved, many of which have unknown functions (Michel 2005). This lack of complete understanding adds another layer of complexity when interpreting the results of different genetic knockout models and their impact on fluoroquinolone resistance and bacterial adaptation.

Conclusion

Methodological differences on key aspects of FQ research complicate the interpretation and comparison of results. These inconsistencies extend to fundamental aspects of FQ activity, including their drug-specific interactions with bacterial DNA gyrase and topoisomerase IV, as well as the variability in resistance development among bacterial species. The influence of FQ structure on binding affinities, the drug-specific stabilization of gyrase-DNA cleavage complexes, and the role of persister cell formation further emphasize the need for more detailed understanding of the mechanisms underlying differential efficacy and resistance.

References

Aedo S, Tse-Dinh YC (2012) Isolation and quantitation of topoisomerase complexes accumulated on Escherichia coli chromosomal DNA. Antimicrob Agents Chemother 56(11):5458–5464. https://doi.org/10.1128/AAC.01182-12. Epub 2012 Aug 6. PMID: 22869559; PMCID: PMC3486612

Alam MK, Alhhazmi A, DeCoteau JF, Luo Y, Geyer CR (2016) RecA inhibitors potentiate antibiotic activity and block evolution of antibiotic resistance. Cell Chem Biol 23(3):381–391. https://doi.org/10.1016/j.chembiol.2016.02.010

Aminimanizani A, Beringer P, Jelliffe R (2001) Comparative pharmacokinetics and pharmacodynamics of the newer fluoroquinolone antibacterials. Clin Pharmacokinet 40(3):169–187. https://doi.org/10.2165/00003088-200140030-00003

Ball P (2000) Moxifloxacin (Avelox): an 8-methoxyquinolone antibacterial with enhanced potency. Int J Clin Pract 54(5):329–332

Beaber JW, Hochhut B, Waldor MK (2004) SOS response promotes horizontal dissemination of antibiotic resistance genes. Nature 427(6969):72–74. https://doi.org/10.1038/nature02241. Epub 2003 Dec 21

Bhatt S, Chatterjee S (2022) Fluoroquinolone antibiotics: occurrence, mode of action, resistance, environmental detection, and remediation—a comprehensive review. Environ Pollut 315:120440. https://doi.org/10.1016/j.envpol.2022.120440. Epub 2022 Oct 17

Briales A, Rodriguez-Martinez JM, Velasco C, Machuca J, Díaz de Alba P, Blazquez J, Pascual A (2012) Exposure to diverse antimicrobials induces the expression of qnrB1, qnrD and smaqnr genes by SOS-dependent regulation. J Antimicrob Chemother 67(12):2854–2859. https://doi.org/10.1093/jac/dks326. Epub 2012 Aug 22

Brighty KE, Gootz TD (1997) Activity of quinolones against other topoisomerases. J Antimicrob Chemother 39(Suppl. B):1–14

Brighty KE, Gootz TD (2000) Chapter 2—Chemistry and mechanism of action of the Quinolone antibacterials. In: The Quinolones, 3rd edn, pp 33–97. https://doi.org/10.1016/B978-012059517-4/50003-9

Bryskier A (1993) Fluoroquinolones: mechanisms of action and resistance. Int J Antimicrob Agents 2(3):151–183. https://doi.org/10.1016/0924-8579(93)90052-7

Bunnell BE, Escobar JF, Bair KL, Sutton MD, Crane JK (2017) Zinc blocks SOS-induced antibiotic resistance via inhibition of RecA in Escherichia coli. PLoS One 12(5):e0178303. https://doi.org/10.1371/journal.pone.0178303. PMID: 28542496; PMCID: PMC5440055

Bush NG, Diez-Santos I, Abbott LR, Maxwell A (2020) Quinolones: mechanism, lethality and their contributions to antibiotic resistance. Molecules 25(23):5662. https://doi.org/10.3390/molecules25235662. PMID: 33271787; PMCID: PMC7730664

Chen CR, Malik M, Snyder M, Drlica K (1996) DNA gyrase and topoisomerase IV on the bacterial chromosome: quinolone-induced DNA cleavage. J Mol Biol 258(4):627–637. https://doi.org/10.1006/jmbi.1996.0274

Cirz RT, Chin JK, Andes DR, de Crécy-Lagard V, Craig WA, Romesberg FE (2005) Inhibition of mutation and combating the evolution of antibiotic resistance. PLoS Biol 3(6):e176. https://doi.org/10.1371/journal.pbio.0030176. Epub 2005 May 10. PMID: 15869329; PMCID: PMC1088971

Da Re S, Garnier F, Guérin E, Campoy S, Denis F, Ploy MC (2009) The SOS response promotes qnrB quinolone-resistance determinant expression. EMBO Rep 10(8):929–933. https://doi.org/10.1038/embor.2009.99. Epub 2009 Jun 26. PMID: 19556999; PMCID: PMC2726673

Da Silva Ribeiro AC, da Silva Martins WMB, Aderito da Silva A, Gales AC, Galasse Rando DG, da Rocha Minarin LA (2020) Exposure to sub-inhibitory ciprofloxacin and nitrofurantoin concentrations increases recA gene expression in uropathogenic Escherichia coli: the role of RecA protein as a drug target. Eur J Pharm Sci 146:105268. https://doi.org/10.1016/j.ejps.2020.105268. ISSN 0928-0987

Dalhoff A (2012) Global fluoroquinolone resistance epidemiology and implictions for clinical use. Interdiscip Perspect Infect Dis 2012:976273. https://doi.org/10.1155/2012/976273. Epub 2012 Oct 14. PMID: 23097666; PMCID: PMC3477668

Denis A, Moreau NJ (1993) Mechanisms of quinolone resistance in clinical isolates: accumulation of sparfloxacin and of fluoroquinolones of various hydrophobicity, and analysis of membrane composition. J Antimicrob Chemother 32(3):379–392. https://doi.org/10.1093/jac/32.3.379

Diaz-Diaz S, Recacha E, Machuca J, García-Duque A, Docobo-Pérez F, Blázquez J, Pascual A, Rodríguez-Martínez JM (2021) Synergistic quinolone sensitization by targeting the recA SOS response gene and oxidative stress. Antimicrob Agents Chemother 65(4):e02004–e02020. https://doi.org/10.1128/AAC.02004-20. PMID: 33526493; PMCID: PMC8097469

Domagala JM (1994) Structure-activity and structure-side-effect relationships for the quinolone antibacterials. J Antimicrob Chemother 33(4):685–706. https://doi.org/10.1093/jac/33.4.685. Erratum in: J Antimicrob Chemother 1994 Nov;34(5):851

Drlica K, Malik M, Kerns RJ, Zhao X (2008) Quinolone-mediated bacterial death. Antimicrob Agents Chemother 52(2):385–392. https://doi.org/10.1128/AAC.01617-06. Epub 2007 Aug 27. PMID: 17724149; PMCID: PMC2224783

EMA (2023) Fluoroquinolone antibiotics reminder measures reduce risk long long-lasting disabling and potentially irreversible side effects. Available from: https://www.ema.europa.eu/en/news/fluoroquinolone-antibiotics-reminder-measures-reduce-risk-long-lasting-disabling-and-potentially-irreversible-side-effects

File TM Jr (1999) Overview of resistance in the 1990s. Chest 115(3 Suppl):3S–8S. https://doi.org/10.1378/chest.115.suppl_1.3s

Fournier B, Zhao X, Lu T, Drlica K, Hooper DC (2000) Selective targeting of topoisomerase IV and DNA gyrase in Staphylococcus aureus: different patterns of quinolone-induced inhibition of DNA synthesis. Antimicrob Agents Chemother 44(8):2160–2165. https://doi.org/10.1128/AAC.44.8.2160-2165.2000. PMID: 10898691; PMCID: PMC90029

Fukuda H, Hiramatsu K (1999) Primary targets of fluoroquinolones in Streptococcus pneumoniae. Antimicrob Agents Chemother 43(2):410–412. https://doi.org/10.1128/AAC.43.2.410. PMID: 9925547; PMCID: PMC89092

Goossens H, Sprenger MJ (1998) Community acquired infections and bacterial resistance. BMJ 317(7159):654–657. https://doi.org/10.1136/bmj.317.7159.654. PMID: 9727998; PMCID: PMC1113837

Higgins PG, Fluit AC, Schmitz FJ (2003) Fluoroquinolones: structure and target sites. Curr Drug Targets 4(2):181–190. https://doi.org/10.2174/1389450033346920

Hooper DC (1998) Clinical applications of quinolones. Biochim Biophys Acta Gene Struct Expr 1400(1–3):45–61. ISSN 0167-4781. https://doi.org/10.1016/S0167-4781(98)00127-4

Hooper DC (1999) Mode of action of fluoroquinolones. Drugs 58(Suppl 2):6–10. https://doi.org/10.2165/00003495-199958002-00002

Hooper DC (2001) Mechanisms of action of antimicrobials: focus on fluoroquinolones. Clin Infect Dis 32(Suppl 1):S9–S15. https://doi.org/10.1086/319370

Jacoby GA, Corcoran MA, Hooper DC (2015) Protective effect of Qnr on agents other than quinolones that target DNA gyrase. Antimicrob Agents Chemother 59(11):6689–6695. https://doi.org/10.1128/AAC.01292-15. Epub 2015 Aug 3. PMID: 26239981; PMCID: PMC4604369

Janion C (2008) Inducible SOS response system of DNA repair and mutagenesis in Escherichia coli. Int J Biol Sci 4(6):338–344. https://doi.org/10.7150/ijbs.4.338. PMID: 18825275; PMCID: PMC2556049

Jaramillo-Riveri S, Broughton J, McVey A, Pilizota T, Scott M, El Karoui M (2022) Growth-dependent heterogeneity in the DNA damage response in Escherichia coli. Mol Syst Biol 18(5):e10441. https://doi.org/10.15252/msb.202110441. PMID: 35620827; PMCID: PMC9136515

Khodursky AB, Zechiedrich EL, Cozzarelli NR (1995) Topoisomerase IV is a target of quinolones in Escherichia coli. Proc Natl Acad Sci USA 92(25):11801–11805. https://doi.org/10.1073/pnas.92.25.11801. PMID: 8524852; PMCID: PMC40490

Madurga S, Sánchez-Céspedes J, Belda I, Vila J, Giralt E (2008) Mechanism of binding of fluoroquinolones to the quinolone resistance-determining region of DNA gyrase: towards an understanding of the molecular basis of quinolone resistance. Chembiochem 9(13):2081–2086. https://doi.org/10.1002/cbic.200800041

Maslowska KH, Makiela-Dzbenska K, Fijalkowska IJ (2019) The SOS system: a complex and tightly regulated response to DNA damage. Environ Mol Mutagen 60(4):368–384. https://doi.org/10.1002/em.22267. Epub 2019 Jan 7. PMID: 30447030; PMCID: PMC6590174

Maso L, Vascon F, Chinellato M, Goormaghtigh F, Bellio P, Campagnaro E, Van Melderen L, Ruzzene M, Pardon E, Angelini A, Celenza G, Steyaert J, Tondi D, Cendron L (2022) Nanobodies targeting LexA autocleavage disclose a novel suppression strategy of SOS-response pathway. Structure 30(11):1479–1493.e9. https://doi.org/10.1016/j.str.2022.09.004. Epub 2022 Oct 13

Michel B (2005) After 30 years of study, the bacterial SOS response still surprises us. PLoS Biol 3(7):e255. https://doi.org/10.1371/journal.pbio.0030255. Epub 2005 Jul 12. PMID: 16000023; PMCID: PMC1174825

Mo CY, Manning SA, Roggiani M, Culyba MJ, Samuels AN, Sniegowski PD, Goulian M, Kohli RM (2016) Systematically altering bacterial SOS activity under stress reveals therapeutic strategies for potentiating antibiotics. mSphere 1(4):e00163–e00116. https://doi.org/10.1128/mSphere.00163-16. PMID: 27536734; PMCID: PMC4980697

Naeem A, Badshah SL, Muska M, Ahmad N, Khan K (2016) The current case of quinolones: synthetic approaches and antibacterial activity. Molecules 21(4):268. https://doi.org/10.3390/molecules21040268. PMID: 27043501; PMCID: PMC6274096

Ojkic N, Lilja E, Direito S, Dawson A, Allen RJ, Waclaw B (2020) A roadblock-and-kill mechanism of action model for the DNA-targeting antibiotic ciprofloxacin. Antimicrob Agents Chemother 64(9):e02487–e02419. https://doi.org/10.1128/AAC.02487-19. PMID: 32601161; PMCID: PMC7449190

Pan XS, Fisher LM (1997) Targeting of DNA gyrase in Streptococcus pneumoniae by sparfloxacin: selective targeting of gyrase or topoisomerase IV by quinolones. Antimicrob Agents Chemother 41(2):471–474. https://doi.org/10.1128/AAC.41.2.471. PMID: 9021211; PMCID: PMC163733

Pan XS, Fisher LM (1998) DNA gyrase and topoisomerase IV are dual targets of clinafloxacin action in Streptococcus pneumoniae. Antimicrob Agents Chemother 42(11):2810–2816. https://doi.org/10.1128/AAC.42.11.2810. PMID: 9797208; PMCID: PMC105948

Pan XS, Ambler J, Mehtar S, Fisher LM (1996) Involvement of topoisomerase IV and DNA gyrase as ciprofloxacin targets in Streptococcus pneumoniae. Antimicrob Agents Chemother 40(10):2321–2326. https://doi.org/10.1128/AAC.40.10.2321. PMID: 8891138; PMCID: PMC163528

Pestova E, Millichap JJ, Noskin GA, Peterson LR (2000) Intracellular targets of moxifloxacin: a comparison with other fluoroquinolones. J Antimicrob Chemother 45(5):583–590. https://doi.org/10.1093/jac/45.5.583

Pham TDM, Ziora ZM, Blaskovich MAT (2019) Quinolone antibiotics. Medchemcomm 10(10):1719–1739. https://doi.org/10.1039/c9md00120d. PMID: 31803393; PMCID: PMC6836748

Piddock LJ, Jin YF, Griggs DJ (2001) Effect of hydrophobicity and molecular mass on the accumulation of fluoroquinolones by Staphylococcus aureus. J Antimicrob Chemother 47(3):261–270. https://doi.org/10.1093/jac/47.3.261

Recacha E, Machuca J, Díaz de Alba P, Ramos-Güelfo M, Docobo-Pérez F, Rodriguez-Beltrán J, Blázquez J, Pascual A, Rodríguez-Martínez JM (2017) Quinolone resistance reversion by targeting the SOS response. MBio 8(5):e00971–e00917. https://doi.org/10.1128/mBio.00971-17. PMID: 29018116; PMCID: PMC5635686

Recacha E, Machuca J, Díaz-Díaz S, García-Duque A, Ramos-Guelfo M, Docobo-Pérez F, Blázquez J, Pascual A, Rodríguez-Martínez JM (2019) Suppression of the SOS response modifies spatiotemporal evolution, post-antibiotic effect, bacterial fitness and biofilm formation in quinolone-resistant Escherichia coli. J Antimicrob Chemother 74(1):66–73. https://doi.org/10.1093/jac/dky407

Rosendahl I, Siemens J, Kindler R, Groeneweg J, Zimmermann J, Czerwinski S, Lamshöft M, Laabs V, Wilke BM, Vereecken H, Amelung W (2012) Persistence of the fluoroquinolone antibiotic difloxacin in soil and lacking effects on nitrogen turnover. J Environ Qual 41(4):1275–1283. https://doi.org/10.2134/jeq2011.0459

Rusu A, Hancu G, Uivaroşi V (2015) Fluoroquinolone pollution of food, water and soil, and bacterial resistance. Environ Chem Lett 13:21–36. https://doi.org/10.1007/s10311-014-0481-3

Schedletzky H, Wiedemann B, Heisig P (1999) The effect of moxifloxacin on its target topoisomerases from Escherichia coli and Staphylococcus aureus. J Antimicrob Chemother 43(Suppl B):31–37. https://doi.org/10.1093/jac/43.suppl_2.31

Selwood T, Larsen BJ, Mo CY, Culyba MJ, Hostetler ZM, Kohli RM, Reitz AB, Baugh SDP (2018) Advancement of the 5-Amino-1-(Carbamoylmethyl)-1H-1,2,3-Triazole-4-Carboxamide Scaffold to disarm the bacterial SOS response. Front Microbiol 9:2961. https://doi.org/10.3389/fmicb.2018.02961. PMID: 30619111; PMCID: PMC6305444

Singh R, Ledesma KR, Chang KT, Tam VH (2010) Impact of recA on levofloxacin exposure-related resistance development. Antimicrob Agents Chemother 54(10):4262–4268. https://doi.org/10.1128/AAC.00168-10. Epub 2010 Jul 26. PMID: 20660686; PMCID: PMC2944593

Tang J, Brynildsen MP (2023) Genome-wide mapping of fluoroquinolone-stabilized DNA gyrase cleavage sites displays drug specific effects that correlate with bacterial persistence. Nucleic Acids Res 51(3):1208–1228. https://doi.org/10.1093/nar/gkac1223. PMID: 36631985; PMCID: PMC9943676

Teichmann L, Luitwieler S, Bengtsson-Palme J, ter Kuile BH (2025) Fluoroquinolone-specific resistance trajectories in E. coli and their dependence on the SOS-response. BMC Microbiol 25:37. https://doi.org/10.1186/s12866-025-03771-5

Thi TD, López E, Rodríguez-Rojas A, Rodríguez-Beltrán J, Couce A, Guelfo JR, Castañeda-García A, Blázquez J (2011) Effect of recA inactivation on mutagenesis of Escherichia coli exposed to sublethal concentrations of antimicrobials. J Antimicrob Chemother 66(3):531–538. https://doi.org/10.1093/jac/dkq496. Epub 2011 Jan 5

Torres-Barceló C, Kojadinovic M, Moxon R, MacLean RC (2015) The SOS response increases bacterial fitness, but not evolvability, under a sublethal dose of antibiotic. Proc Biol Sci 282(1816):20150885. https://doi.org/10.1098/rspb.2015.0885. PMID: 26446807; PMCID: PMC4614765

Tran JH, Jacoby GA, Hooper DC (2005) Interaction of the plasmid-encoded quinolone resistance protein Qnr with Escherichia coli DNA gyrase. Antimicrob Agents Chemother 49(1):118–125. https://doi.org/10.1128/AAC.49.1.118-125.2005. PMID: 15616284; PMCID: PMC538914

Urios A, Herrera G, Aleixandre V, Blanco M (1991) Influence of recA mutations on gyrA dependent quinolone resistance. Biochimie 73(4):519–521. https://doi.org/10.1016/0300-9084(91)90123-i

Van Doorslaer X, Dewulf J, Van Langenhove H, Demeestere K (2014) Fluoroquinolone antibiotics: an emerging class of environmental micropollutants. Sci Total Environ 500-501:250–269. https://doi.org/10.1016/j.scitotenv.2014.08.075. Epub 2014 Sep 16

Vestergaard M, Paulander W, Ingmer H (2015) Activation of the SOS response increases the frequency of small colony variants. BMC Res Notes 8:749. https://doi.org/10.1186/s13104-015-1735-2. PMID: 26643526; PMCID: PMC4672542

Walker GC (1996) The SOS response of Escherichia coli. E coli Salmonella Cell Mol Biol 1(2):1400–1416

Williams AB (2014) Spontaneous mutation rates come into focus in Escherichia coli. DNA Repair (Amst) 24:73–79. https://doi.org/10.1016/j.dnarep.2014.09.009. Epub 2014 Oct 11

World Health Organization (2019) WHO consolidated guidelines on drug-resistant tuberculosis treatment. Available from: https://www.who.int/publications/i/item/9789241550529

Wright DH, Brown GH, Peterson ML, Rotschafer JC (2000) Application of fluoroquinolone pharmacodynamics. J Antimicrob Chemother 46(5):669–683. https://doi.org/10.1093/jac/46.5.669

Zhanel GG, Walkty A, Vercaigne L, Karlowsky JA, Embil J, Gin AS, Hoban DJ (1999) The new fluoroquinolones: a critical review. Can J Infect Dis 10(3):207–238. https://doi.org/10.1155/1999/378394. PMID: 22346384; PMCID: PMC3250697

Chapter 6
EU Laws and Regulations as an Example of Rules for the Veterinary Application of Antimicrobials

Benno ter Kuile

Abstract The most detailed legislation on veterinary antimicrobials and their application for livestock has been adopted by the EU. The consequences of this legislation for daily practice and the effects on development and spreading of resistance are considerable. Monitoring remains an important part of the duties of the competent authorities. The legislation reflects the scientific insights of the time on how to prevent avoidable resistance. Preventing exposure of bacteria to non-lethal concentrations of antimicrobials is a main purpose. The regulations EU 2019/4/5/6 provide the member states with legal tools to enforce good practice and prudent use with regard to the veterinary application of antibiotics.

Keywords EU legislation on AMR · Competent authority · Good practice · Prudent use · Veterinary application of antibiotics

Introduction

In the previous chapters many aspects of usage of antibiotics for veterinary health care have been discussed. In this chapter the Regulations EU 2019/4, 2019/5 and 2019/6 of the European Union will be examined as examples of rules and regulations aiming to limit the negative consequences of the use of antimicrobials. One of the main aims of these three regulations was to implement the scientific consensus of the moment drafting. As is specifically stated in the considerations of the "Veterinary Medicines Regulation" EU 2019/6 "the regulatory framework for

B. ter Kuile (✉)
Department of Molecular Biology and Microbial Food Safety, Swammerdam Institute of Life Sciences, University of Amsterdam, Amsterdam, and the Netherlands Food and Consumer Products Safety Authority, Utrecht, The Netherlands
e-mail: b.h.terkuile@uva.nl

B. ter Kuile (ed.), *Antimicrobial Resistance and Antibiotics Usage in Livestock*,
https://doi.org/10.1007/978-3-032-04598-0_6

veterinary medicinal products should be adapted to scientific progress". Therefore it is useful to scrutinize to which extent the indeed succeed to convert the scientific insights into effective legislation.

Estimates of the amounts of antimicrobials used for livestock in comparison to humans vary widely, but it is highly likely that more is used for animals (Cully 2014). The comparison in weight of active compounds may not be entirely valid, but if used as an indication, in the EU 62% in tons is for livestock and 38% for humans (EFSA/ECDC 2024a, b). The effect of veterinary usage on resistance encountered in human health care is best evaluated with the "One Health" framework (Collignon et al. 2016; Queenan et al. 2016; Collignon and McEwen 2019). The EU reports on application of antibiotics and incidence of resistance, such as the Joint Interagency Antimicrobial Consumption and Resistance Analysis (JIACRA) Reports (ECDC et al. 2017; EFSA/ECDC 2024a, 2024b), are invariably written from a One Health perspective. These principles have recently been translated into proposals for concrete measures (Horvat and Kovacevic 2025). The knowledge, insights and information of the previous chapters will be used in this concluding chapter to provide further recommendations for the application of antimicrobials for animal health and welfare.

It is generally recognized that exposure to non-lethal concentrations of antibiotics forms the greatest risk for development and spreading of resistance (Ter Kuile et al. 2016; Llewelyn et al. 2017). Exposure to concentrations that allow bacteria to survive and adapt is almost unavoidable on farms when antibiotics are mixed into the feed or the drinking water. In both cases not all animals receive equal doses and some will not receive enough to achieve the so-called "area under the curve", a term used in pharmacodynamics to indicate the time bacteria are exposed to levels exceeding the minimal inhibitory concentration (MIC) (Lv and Wang 2024). Development of resistance already occurs during exposure to low concentrations of antimicrobials, in the case of fluoroquinolones as low as 1% of the MIC (Gullberg et al. 2011). For most other antibiotics the threshold is higher, by at 10% of the MIC development and selection of resistance take place (Andersson and Hughes 2014; Hughes 2014). Since leftovers of antimicrobials frequently end up in water, development of and selection for antibiotic resistance often occurs in aquatic environments (Miranda et al. 2022).

Policy Aims and Potential Measures to Reduce the Effects of Usage of Antibiotics in Livestock

When formulating proposals for measures and designing policies for reducing the effects of veterinary applications of antimicrobials, a balance must be found between the benefits for public health and the costs in terms of animal health and welfare and extra expenses for farmers. On the one hand, forcing farmers to implement expensive measures is of little use if the corresponding gains in public health are minimal.

On the other hand, antimicrobial resistance is a cost factor at farms as well (Lhermie et al. 2018a, b). Animals remain diseased for longer times, infections keep on spreading, and treatment becomes more expensive. For these reasons the agricultural sector has an interest in preventing development and spreading of resistance. With the presently available information, it is hard to quantify the financial interest of the veterinary sector as a whole. It is clear, however, that not being able to use antimicrobials to treat infections in livestock would be very costly for this sector (Horvat and Kovacevic 2025).

The aim of veterinary treatment protocols is to clear infections in livestock without causing unnecessary side-effects with respect to resistance. The so-called "prudent-use" guidelines are drafted with this aim in mind (Sucena Afonso et al. 2024). The application of antimicrobials as growth promotors is particularly harmful, as this caused exposure to low concentrations of antibiotics. Within the EU this practice has been banned since 2006. This ban, in combination with other measures, has lead initially to stabilization of the levels of resistance, followed by a gradual decrease in some of the EU member states (EFSA/ECDC 2024a, b). In most member states the low hanging fruits have been picked, and further random reduction of antibiotic use could be harmful for animal health and welfare. Therefore, after this general reduction, specific measures, such as improved dosing methodology, should be used to achieve the therapeutic goals while limiting development and spreading of resistance. In addition measures aiming to reduce the chance of infections might even be more effective.

The reduction of antibiotic usage for livestock by almost 70% in The Netherlands in the period 2009–2019 (Heederik 2020), has resulted in measurable reductions of resistance in the microbiota of food production animals (Veldman et al. 2020, 2024). A reduction that sometimes exceeded 50% was observed in indicator *E. coli* from varying sources when values form 2018 were compared to those of the years 2007–2011. Probably more important is the synchronous reduction of resistance in humans *Salmonella* isolates. Human *Salmonella* infections are mostly foodborne (Pires et al. 2014) and the treatment protocols for human infections were not changed during that period. This indicates that the reduction in resistance is at least partially related to the reduced veterinary antibiotic usage.

The degree in which exposure to non-lethal concentrations of antibiotics causes development and spread of resistance depends on the length and frequency of that exposure (Andersson and Hughes 2014). Reduction of usage by lowering the dose would be a very dangerous way to try to achieve a statistical reduction, as it would cause more rather than less resistance by exposing bacteria to non-lethal concentrations. The optimal treatment strategy could be phrased as "the highest dose the patient (human or animal) can handle for the shortest time needed to clear the infection" (Llewelyn et al. 2017; Ramasco et al. 2024). Unfortunately, this may conflict with the instructions for usage supplied by the manufacturer. These instructions are written in consultation with the competent authority and are part of the of the authorization procedures allowing to market the product for the specifically described purposes. Veterinarians legally are not allowed to ignore these instructions. This causes the unwanted situation that a veterinarian may not be in compliance with the law when she/he proscribes the optimal dosing protocol. Hence, it should be made legally possible for a prescribing veterinarian to deviate from the instructions of the manufacturer, with a well-motivated alternative that optimizes antibiotic use in particular cases.

It is quite possible that at a certain stage further reduction of veterinary antibiotic use will be incompatible with animal health and welfare (Ferri et al. 2017; de Jong et al. 2023). When, in order to reduce the total amount of antibiotics used, treatment against an infection is withheld from an animals, it will suffer unnecessarily. The overall aim of reducing the resistance originally selected in the agricultural sector that ends up in the human health care sector, must be achieved by carefully designed policies. Not treating or treating with insufficient doses, increases the risks of transfer of resistance for livestock to humans (Stegeman and Schakenraad 2016). There are three options to prevent development and spreading of resistance:

1. Preventing infections by improving hygiene and keeping facilities clean
2. Protection of the animals by means of vaccination programs
3. Improving treatment protocols so that the infection is cleared with minimal resistance development.

The prevention of exposing bacteria to sublethal concentrations can in addition be achieved by avoiding carry over during manufacturing of medicated feed, leakage of antibiotics from farms, and pre-treatment of feces use a fertilizer or other ways of disposal.

Present Practice Using Antimicrobials on Poultry, Pigs and Meat Calves

In many EU member states prescribing antimicrobials is licensed solely to veterinarians. The farmers can subsequently store and administer the prescribed antibiotics on his farm. Some member states require farms to have a "company health plan", "farm treatment plan" or a comparable document in which the farmer and the veterinarian describe the diseases most often observed and the treatment prescribed in those cases. This type of plan is an effective tool to protect public health at a limited administrative burden, as stated in the fifth consideration of EU 2019/6. In addition, formularies are drafted by professional organizations and approved by competent authorities. These formularies provide lists of medicines, including antimicrobial agents, that have been approved by that authority for use on farms. A formulary will give a list of first choice, and less desirable antibiotics as second and third and sometimes even fourth choice for a specific illness in a particular animal species. First choice antibiotics are effective and have limited risks of resistance development. Hence they can be part of the abovementioned farm treatment plans. Second choice medicines can only be applied when a clearly documented need to do so exists. Third choice drugs are usually reserved for human usage and may only be used on individual animals after a microbiological test shows that due to resistance this is the only effective antibiotic available. The prescribing veterinarian is responsible for complying with the law. In some case it would be best both for the treatment and from the viewpoint of avoiding resistance to deviate from the formulary or the manufacturer's instructions. Presently the law does not provide that possibility.

WHO has a list of "highest priority critically important antimicrobials" to be preserved for human usage (Collignon et al. 2016; Lhermie et al. 2020). These antibiotics may only in exceptional cases and under very strict conditions be used for livestock. Every few years this list is updated based on the most recent antimicrobial resistance monitoring data. A comparable and even more detailed list has been drawn up by the European Medicines Agency (EMA) (EMA 2019). The present lists reserve the quinolones, third and higher generation cephalosporins, macrolides, glycopeptides, ketolides, and polymyxins for human usage and thus ban them from veterinary use. Some antibiotics from these classes are explicitly reserved for veterinary application. The antibiotics reserved for human use may only be used as third choice, and thus a means of last resort, for livestock. The EU reserves the right to deviate from the WHO lists, but rarely does that and if so only on details.

It is not unusual for veterinarians to not only prescribe medicines, but to also sell them to the farms they are responsible for. This creates a conflict of interests, as the vet does profit financially from prescribing antibiotics. Whether or not financial considerations play any role in the decision to apply antimicrobials, there will always be a semblance of a conflict of interests. Therefore it is useful to monitor the prescription records of individual veterinarians, so that those individuals that prescribe more than their colleagues can be identified and asked to explain their prescriptions. This monitoring is obligatory according to EU 2019/6 article 57.

Application Methodologies

Broilers and laying hens always receive any necessary antimicrobials as group treatment. Poultry most receives antibiotic through the drinking water. To do that the dosing system is connected to the drinking water supply. Sick birds drink less than healthy animals, so they receive less antibiotics while they need more. The overall outcome is underdosing of the sick animals and overdosing of their healthy counterparts. Another major problem of distributing the antibiotics through the water is that drug may precipitate on the inside of the tubes. These deposits can redissolve later, resulting in an extended exposure to low levels of antibiotics. If during an inspection of the system water samples are taken that turn out to contain antimicrobials, it cannot be ascertained whether these were illegally added as growth promoter, or were the left-overs from a legitimate treatment. The problems caused by the initial precipitation can be avoided by properly rinsing the water system after treatment. This, however, is time consuming for the farmer and adherence to the correct procedures will have to be enforced.

Pigs can receive antibiotics through medicated water or feed, by top-dressing feed, or through injection. The use of a repeat-dosing injection gun has shown to be a very effective manner to apply antibiotics to pigs and piglets. This way of application is by far better from the viewpoint of preventing resistance development than the other systems, because each animals receives the correct dose, no leftovers can contaminate the environment and the microbiota of the intestines are less exposed to the antibiotics. Medicated feed has the problem of carry-over when afterwards non-medicated feed is manufactured on the same production line and top-dressing results in uneven distribution. Since the injection with repeat-dosing guns has been shown to be feasible, also on a comparatively large scale, this method is to be preferred over the others.

Meat calves are known antibiotic users (Cheng et al. 2024). In contrast, for on dairy farms antimicrobial therapy is mostly limited to the dry-off period for lactating cows (Abdelfattah et al. 2024). Milk of cows treated with antibiotics is not allowed to be marketed and this generates considerable costs for farmers. This strongly reduces the amount of antimicrobials used on dairy cows. Meat calves are transported at a very young age and after transport they often are infected with pathogens, necessitating antimicrobial treatment (Gonzalez et al. 2022). Meat calves mixed during transport and after arrival at the veal farms where they will be raised often exchange pathogens (Marcato et al. 2018). Furthermore, the immune systems of very young calves are not yet sufficiently developed to counter infections without antimicrobials (Siddiqui et al. 2012). As a consequence, antibiotic treatment is often needed after arrival of the young animals at a veal farm (Marcato et al. 2022). The resulting high antibiotic usage may be the unavoidable effect of the practice to remove calves immediately from their mothers and to transport them at a very young age (Marcato et al. 2018).

Measures to Reduce the Need for Applying Antimicrobials

The consideration 4 of the regulation EU 2019/4 states: "*Prevention of disease is better than cure. Medicinal treatments, especially with antimicrobials, should never replace good husbandry, bio-security and management practices*". Article 107, paragraph 1 of the regulation EU 2019/6 prohibits that type of use: "*Antimicrobial medicinal products shall not be applied routinely nor used to compensate for poor hygiene, inadequate animal husbandry or lack of care or to compensate for poor farm management*". This explicit ban provides law enforcement agencies with the tools needed to interfere at the level of farm management and to demand proper hygiene and other good practices in the framework of antimicrobial resistance. The problem is that these are open standards. How is proper hygiene defined? What farm practices and procedures are acceptable and what not? It is up to the law enforcement agencies to provide guidelines that farms will have to stick to.

In the framework of antibiotic resistance, bad hygiene means exposure to large number of microorganisms, among which pathogenic bacteria (Collignon and

McEwen 2019; Kerek et al. 2025). Low air quality and insufficient ventilation can expose the lungs of livestock to pathogenic microbes, causing a risk for airway infections (Roland et al. 2016; Sanz-Fernandez et al. 2023). Airway infections are a common reason for the application of antimicrobials for all livestock that is held inside stables, barns or sheds. The quality of the air is sufficient and the ventilation is adequate when the animals do not develop unnecessary airway infections due to low quality air. Frequent checking of the functioning of automated ventilation systems in animal holdings can improve air quality and thereby contribute to animal health (Schnyder et al. 2019). At present there are no criteria for air quality. These should be formulated in units of microbes or pathogens per cubic meter.

Dirt in animal facilities causes infection and infections reduce growth (Strauch 1991) and animal welfare (Van der Meer 2017). Insufficient hygiene is also a cause of mastitis in dairy cows (Visser et al. 2015; Ruegg 2017). Good hygiene can therefore be described as the state of cleanliness in which no, or at least as little as possible, avoidable infections are caused by manure or other dirt or filth in the surroundings of the animals. Regular removal of manure and other organic materials in which pathogens can reside and multiply is labor intensive. Calculations will have to show which cleaning and disinfection procedures generate enough gain for public health to justify the costs. The design of new animal facilities will have to account the need to easily clean them and preferably prevent the accumulation of dirt. This can be done by avoiding ledges and ridges, having smooth and easy to clean wall covering, etc. floor must compromise between easiness of cleaning and preventing sliding.

"Inadequate animal husbandry" is an even more vague notion, because it comprises a variety of aspects of farm management. Low quality feed contaminated with pathogenic bacteria is a clear risk factor in this category (Davies et al. 2004; Herrero et al. 2023). *Salmonella* often enters the farms through contaminated feed, infects the animals and subsequently remains in the manure (Wilhelm et al. 2012). The presence of *Campylobacter* is usually the result of poor hygiene in the facilities (Nather et al. 2009). There are no microbiological criteria or other legal instrument limiting the presence of *Salmonella* in feed. Possibly this type of enforcement tools can be useful for reducing the risks of exposure, thereby reducing the need for antimicrobial treatments. Monitoring the presence of undesirable microbes in feed could be a first step.

Lack of care and mismanagement are of a heavier category than bad hygiene or inadequate animal husbandry. Lack of care harms animal health and welfare. Law enforcement can and should demand improvements when this is noticed. Mismanagement is a general term that describes a situation one step worse than inadequate management. Immediate action is required in the first case, while in the latter a more moderate response can be sufficient. In those cases the usage of antimicrobials is a minor concern and certainly not the main point of interest.

Which measures in the area of farm management and hygiene can a law enforcement agency demand? This is not straightforwardly described in the Regulation. The policies concerning these matters will have to be formulated in a dialogue between the authorities, law enforcement agencies, the farm sector and the veterinary organizations. This should result in clear and enforceable guidelines. One principle should be that following the advice and instructions of the veterinarian is not optional but an obligation. The kind of measures and investments that can be demanded are specifically relevant for farms that use large amounts of antibiotics over longer periods of time and veterinarians who prescribe more antibiotics than their colleagues with similar practices. The causes can be poor hygiene, bad ventilation, low quality feed or a combination of these and other factors. Addressing these issues will reduce the amount of antimicrobials needed.

Prevention of Transfer of Resistance from Livestock to Human Healthcare

Once resistance has developed and spread in the agricultural sector, it can reach human healthcare in several manners that are not yet fully understood (Mughini-Gras et al. 2019; Hembach et al. 2022). Examples of possible routes are direct animal-human contact, food of animal origin, via soil, air or water or through manure (Huijbers et al. 2015; Medina-Pizzali et al. 2021). Foodstuffs seem a logical route, but are certainly not the only one. Research into the role of surface waters suggested in first instance a role of resistant pathogens in transport of pathogens to the human populations, but follow-up research contradicted that notion (Pallares-Vega et al. 2019). Soil bacteria are rarely sensitive to all antibiotics used in test panels. In one investigation more than 80% of the 412 strains tested were resistant to more than 16 of the 23 antibiotics used in the panels (Walsh and Duffy 2013). Therefore it seems likely that the environment also plays a role in the exchange of resistance between humans and livestock. It is, however, doubtful whether effective measures are possible to prevent this exchange or even just to reduce the magnitude. One of the reasons why it is difficult to reduce the exchange of resistance is that the transfer of resistance is often mediated by plasmids or other agents such as phages and not by intact microbes (Davies and Davies 2010; Partridge et al. 2018).

The transfer of ESBL - *E. coli* from poultry farms to the environment was investigated from the public health point of view (Blaak et al. 2015a, b). The bacteria spread through the air and were also transferred by flies. In addition, increased numbers of viable *E. coli* were measured in the surrounding surface waters shortly after the poultry sheds were cleaned between two rounds of broilers. The water that was used to clean flowed of the terrain into the nearest surface water. This points to a role of the surface waters in spreading microorganisms from farms to the human population. Quantitatively, however, the contribution of farms is considerably less than that of wastewater treatment plants (Pallares-Vega et al. 2019). Manure distributed over the land just before a rain shower caused a short-lasting peak in *E. coli* in surface waters, but otherwise the contribution of agriculture was much limited.

The concentration of antibiotics in milk of cow that are being treated for mastitis is relatively low, but not negligible. This milk must be disposed of in a proper manner. The EFSA opinion "Risk for the development of Antimicrobial Resistance due to feeding of calves with milk containing residues of antibiotics" names a number of possible ways to do this (Ricci et al. 2017), such a fermenting, pH increase, or electrochemical oxidation. Which measures are most effective and implementable still needs to be determined.

In theory countermeasures are possible that would reduce the transfer of resistance from livestock to human health care (Ter Kuile et al. 2016). Nevertheless, it seems unlikely that without considerable research effective measures can be designed that prevent the exchange of resistant microbes after selection for resistance has taken place at the farm. Most likely preventing development and selection to occur in the first place will be more efficient. Potential exceptions are collecting and treating the water used to clean poultry housing and disposing properly of milk from cows treated for mastitis. The positive effects of such measures are hard to quantify and without a proven procedure to achieve this it seems hard to justify demanding measures from farmers. For these reasons research into the implementation of such measures seems desirable.

Monitoring of Antibiotic Resistance and Usage

Since 2014 EU member states have committed themselves to participate in a program for monitoring antimicrobial resistance in microbes from livestock and foodstuffs. Initially the monitoring was prescribed in Implementing Decision 2013/652/EU, later to be updated in Commission Implementing Decision (EU) 2020/1729 on the monitoring and reporting of antimicrobial resistance in zoonotic and commensal bacteria. The implementing decision describes in great detail which samples must be taken and which combinations of bacteria species and antibiotics must be investigated and reported to the EU Commission. Data on usage are not included in this program, but instead prescribed in article 57 paragraph 2 of the regulation 2019/6. That article requires member states to collect data on antibiotic sales and usage. The text of article 57 offers the Commission the possibility to draft an implementing decision of this reporting as well. Paragraph 1 of this same article 57 obliges member states to evaluate the usage at farm level and to report sales per antibiotic and animal species combination to the European Medicines Agency (EMA). The EMA combines and analyses the reports of the member states for an overall report of its own.

Livestock farmers can use benchmark values to compare their antibiotic consumption with that of comparable farms. The aim is that the farms and their veterinarians take action when these benchmarks are exceeded. These benchmarks can furthermore be used to identify veterinarians whose prescription policies need to be corrected. Denmark has for many years been using benchmarks to supervise and correct veterinarians and their experience is that this system reduces the total amount of antibiotics used (Dupont et al. 2017).

Not Covered by the Regulations

The EU regulation 2019 4/5/6 cover production, admission to the market and application of veterinary medicines, including antimicrobials. One aspect of the antibiotic resistance issues is not covered by these regulations: countering certain forms of resistance that are judged particularly hazardous and that occur in the agricultural sector. This does not concern the often occurring forms of resistance against antibiotics that are often used for livestock, but rare forms of resistance against medicines that are critically important for human health care, such as carbapenems and colistin. Resistance against compounds, that are not allowed for veterinary usage can be selected for by usage of other antibiotics, if the genes that cause it are located on the same plasmids as the genes of the antibiotic used for treating the animals. If this occurs at all, it is on single farms. An example of the past was livestock-associated MRSA, selected for by tetracycline usage. In addition, if carbapenem resistant bacteria are found on foodstuffs, measures can only be taken if there is legislation against the specific bacterial species. The resistance alone is no legal ground. Possibly microbiological criteria could be used as legal instrument for such cases, or an emergency risk assessment.

Conclusions

The public health costs for of antimicrobial resistance are in the EU 1.1 Billion Euro per year (Anderson et al. 2023). If indeed, as estimated, about one quarter of all resistance encountered in human health care originates in the veterinary sector (Mughini-Gras et al. 2019), then the costs for public health caused by treating infections in livestock are some 250–300 million euro. Given the total expenses on health care in the EU, not an impressive amount. The costs for the agricultural sector if the use of antimicrobials were completely prohibited would be far higher, and in addition animal health and welfare would be greatly compromised. The reduction of public health costs caused by livestock care can thus only be reduced by better ways of antibiotic application. New vaccines and improved farm management could be instruments to achieve this. In particular exposure of microbes to non-lethal concentrations of antibiotics should be prevented. Therefore, reducing the dose when treatment with antibiotics is needed would be a very dangerous way to reduce the total amount of antimicrobials used. The Eu regulations 2019/4 and 2019/6 form a solid legal basis to enforce good practices with respect to the application of antibiotics. The regulations can mostly be implemented without further interpretation, but some parts are open standards that must be filled in.

References

Abdelfattah EM, Ekong PS, Okello E et al (2024) Antimicrobial drug use and its association with antimicrobial resistance in fecal commensals from cows on California dairies. Front Vet Sci 11:1504640

Anderson M, Panteli D, Mossialos E (2023) How can the EU support sustainable innovation and access to effective antibiotics? Policy options for existing and new medicines. European Observatory on Health Systems and Policies, Copenhagen

Andersson DI, Hughes D (2014) Microbiological effects of sublethal levels of antibiotics. Nat Rev Microbiol 12:465–478

Blaak H, Lynch G, Italiaander R, Hamidjaja RA, Schets FM, de Roda Husman AM (2015a) Multidrug-resistant and extended spectrum beta-lactamase-producing Escherichia coli in Dutch surface water and wastewater. PLoS One 10:e0127752

Blaak H, van Hoek AH, Hamidjaja RA, van der Plaats RQ, Kerkhof-de Heer L, de Roda Husman AM, Schets FM (2015b) Distribution, numbers, and diversity of ESBL-producing E. coli in the Poultry Farm Environment. PloS one 10:e0135402

Cheng TY, Pempek JA, Locke SR, Masterson MA, Habing GG (2024) A survey of antimicrobial use practices on veal farms in the United States. Zoonoses Public Health 71:60–70

Collignon PJ, McEwen SA (2019) One Health-its importance in helping to better control antimicrobial resistance. Trop Med Infect Dis 4(1):22

Collignon PJ, Conly JM, Andremont A et al (2016) World Health Organization ranking of antimicrobials according to their importance in human medicine: a critical step for developing risk management strategies to control antimicrobial resistance from food animal production. Clin Infect Dis 63:1087–1093

Cully M (2014) Public health: the politics of antibiotics. Nature 509:S16–S17

Davies J, Davies D (2010) Origins and evolution of antibiotic resistance. Microbiol Mol Biol Rev 74:417–433

Davies PR, Scott Hurd H, Funk JA, Fedorka-Cray PJ, Jones FT (2004) The role of contaminated feed in the epidemiology and control of Salmonella enterica in pork production. Foodborne Pathog Dis 1:202–215

de Jong E, McCubbin KD, Speksnijder D et al (2023) Invited review: selective treatment of clinical mastitis in dairy cattle. J Dairy Sci 106:3761–3778

Dupont N, Diness LH, Fertner M, Kristensen CS, Stege H (2017) Antimicrobial reduction measures applied in Danish pig herds following the introduction of the "Yellow Card" antimicrobial scheme. Prev Vet Med 138:9–16

ECDC, EFSA & EMA (2017) ECDC/EFSA/EMA second joint report on the integrated analysis of the consumption of antimicrobial agents and occurrence of antimicrobial resistance in bacteria from humans and food-producing animals—Joint Interagency Antimicrobial Consumption and Resistance Analysis (JIACRA) Report. EFSA J 15:135

EFSA/ECDC (2024a) JIACRA 4 Antimicrobial consumption and resistance in bacteria from humans and food-producing animals. EFSA J 172

EFSA/ECDC (2024b) The European Union summary report on antimicrobial resistance in zoonotic and indicator bacteria from humans, animals and food in 2021–2022. pp. 195. EFSA

EMA (2019) Categorisation of antibiotics in the European Union pp. 73. Amsterdam

Ferri M, Ranucci E, Romagnoli P, Giaccone V (2017) Antimicrobial resistance: a global emerging threat to public health systems. Crit Rev Food Sci Nutr 57:2857–2876

Gonzalez TJB, Marcato F, de Freitas CE, van den Brand H, Hoorweg FA, Wolthuis-Fillerup M, Engel B, Schnabel SK, van Reenen CG, Brouwer MSM (2022) Longitudinal study on the prevalence of extended spectrum cephalosporins-resistant Escherichia coli colonization in Dutch veal farms. Vet Microbiol 273:109520

Gullberg E, Cao S, Berg OG, Ilback C, Sandegren L, Hughes D, Andersson DI (2011) Selection of resistant bacteria at very low antibiotic concentrations. PLoS Pathog 7:e1002158

Heederik DJJ (2020) Het gebruik van antibiotica bij landbouwhuisdieren in 2019. pp. 36. Autoriteit Diergeneesmiddelen Utrecht

Hembach N, Bierbaum G, Schreiber C, Schwartz T (2022) Facultative pathogenic bacteria and antibiotic resistance genes in swine livestock manure and clinical wastewater: a molecular biology comparison. Environ Pollut 313:120128

Herrero M, Mason-D'Croz D, Thornton PK, et al. (2023) Livestock and sustainable food systems: status, trends, and priority actions. In: von Braun J, Afsana K, Fresco LO & Hassan MHA (eds) Science and innovations for food systems transformation, Cham (CH), p. 375–399

Horvat O, Kovacevic Z (2025) Human and Veterinary medicine collaboration: synergistic approach to address antimicrobial resistance through the lens of planetary health. Antibiotics (Basel) 14

Hughes D (2014) Selection and evolution of resistance to antimicrobial drugs. IUBMB Life 66:521–529

Huijbers PM, Blaak H, de Jong MC, Graat EA, Vandenbroucke-Grauls CM, de Roda Husman AM (2015) Role of the environment in the transmission of antimicrobial resistance to humans: a review. Environ Sci Technol 49:11993–12004

Kerek A, Roman I, Szabo A, Kovacs D, Kardos G, Kovacs L, Jerzsele A (2025) Antibiotic resistance genes in Escherichia coli - literature review. Crit Rev Microbiol:1–35

Lhermie G, Tauer LW, Grohn YT (2018a) An assessment of the economic costs to the U.S. dairy market of antimicrobial use restrictions. Prev Vet Med 160:63–67

Lhermie G, Tauer LW, Grohn YT (2018b) The farm cost of decreasing antimicrobial use in dairy production. PLoS One 13:e0194832

Lhermie G, La Ragione RM, Weese JS, Olsen JE, Christensen JP, Guardabassi L (2020) Indications for the use of highest priority critically important antimicrobials in the veterinary sector. J Antimicrob Chemother 75:1671–1680

Liu GY, Yu D, Fan MM, Zhang X, Jin ZY, Tang C, Liu XF (2024a) Antimicrobial resistance crisis: could artificial intelligence be the solution? Mil Med Res 11:7

Liu JH, Liu YY, Shen YB, Yang J, Walsh TR, Wang Y, Shen J (2024b) Plasmid-mediated colistin-resistance genes: mcr. Trends Microbiol 32:365–378

Llewelyn MJ, Fitzpatrick JM, Darwin E, Sarah Tonkin C, Gorton C, Paul J, Peto TEA, Yardley L, Hopkins S, Walker AS (2017) The antibiotic course has had its day. BMJ 358:j3418

Lv G, Wang Y (2024) Machine learning-based antibiotic resistance prediction models: an updated systematic review and meta-analysis. Technol Health Care 32:2865–2882

Marcato F, van den Brand H, Kemp B, van Reenen K (2018) Evaluating potential biomarkers of health and performance in veal calves. Front Vet Sci 5:133

Marcato F, van den Brand H, Kemp B, Engel B, Schnabel SK, Hoorweg FA, Wolthuis-Fillerup M, van Reenen K (2022) Effects of transport age and calf and maternal characteristics on health and performance of veal calves. J Dairy Sci 105:1452–1468

Medina-Pizzali ML, Hartinger SM, Salmon-Mulanovich G, Larson A, Riveros M, Mausezahl D (2021) Antimicrobial resistance in rural settings in Latin America: a scoping review with a one health lens. Int J Environ Res Public Health 18

Miranda CD, Concha C, Godoy FA, Lee MR (2022) Aquatic environments as hotspots of transferable low-level quinolone resistance and their potential contribution to high-level quinolone resistance. Antibiotics (Basel) 11

Mughini-Gras L, Dorado-Garcia A, van Duijkeren E et al (2019) Attributable sources of community-acquired carriage of Escherichia coli containing beta-lactam antibiotic resistance genes: a population-based modelling study. Lancet Planet Health 3:e357–e369

Nather G, Alter T, Martin A, Ellerbroek L (2009) Analysis of risk factors for Campylobacter species infection in broiler flocks. Poult Sci 88:1299–1305

Pallares-Vega R, Blaak H, van der Plaats R, de Roda Husman AM, Hernandez Leal L, van Loosdrecht MCM, Weissbrodt DG, Schmitt H (2019) Determinants of presence and removal of antibiotic resistance genes during WWTP treatment: a cross-sectional study. Water Res 161:319–328

Partridge SR, Kwong SM, Firth N, Jensen SO (2018) Mobile genetic elements associated with antimicrobial resistance. Clin Microbiol Rev 31

Pires SM, Vieira AR, Hald T, Cole D (2014) Source attribution of human salmonellosis: an overview of methods and estimates. Foodborne Pathog Dis 11:667–676

Queenan K, Hasler B, Rushton J (2016) A One Health approach to antimicrobial resistance surveillance: is there a business case for it? Int J Antimicrob Agents 48:422–427

Ramasco F, Mendez R, Suarez de la Rica A, Gonzalez de Castro R, Maseda E (2024) Sepsis stewardship: the puzzle of antibiotic therapy in the context of individualization of decision making. J Pers Med 14

Ricci A, Allende A, Bolton D et al (2017) Risk for the development of antimicrobial resistance (AMR) due to feeding of calves with milk containing residues of antibiotics. EFSA J 15

Roland L, Drillich M, Klein-Jobstl D, Iwersen M (2016) Invited review: influence of climatic conditions on the development, performance, and health of calves. J Dairy Sci 99:2438–2452

Ruegg PL (2017) A 100-year review: mastitis detection, management, and prevention. J Dairy Sci 100:10381–10397

Sanz-Fernandez S, Diaz-Gaona C, Borge C, Quintanilla R, Rodriguez-Estevez V (2023) Multi-criteria evaluation model of management for weaned piglets and its relations with farm performance and veterinary medicine consumption. Animals (Basel) 13

Schnyder P, Schonecker L, Schupbach-Regula G, Meylan M (2019) Effects of management practices, animal transport and barn climate on animal health and antimicrobial use in Swiss veal calf operations. Prev Vet Med 167:146–157

Siddiqui N, Price S, Hope J (2012) BCG vaccination of neonatal calves: potential roles for innate immune cells in the induction of protective immunity. Comp Immunol Microbiol Infect Dis 35:219–226

Stegeman JA & Schakenraad MHW (2016) Antibioticabeleid in de Dierhouderij p. 59

Strauch D (1991) Survival of pathogenic micro-organisms and parasites in excreta, manure and sewage sludge. Rev Sci Tech 10:813–846

Sucena Afonso J, El Tholth M, McIntyre KM, Carmo LP, Coyne L, Manriquez D, Raboisson D, Lhermie G, Rushton J (2024) Strategies to reduce antimicrobials in livestock and aquaculture, and their impact under field conditions: a structured scoping literature review. J Antimicrob Chemother 79:11–26

Ter Kuile BH, Kraupner N, Brul S (2016) The risk of low concentrations of antibiotics in agriculture for resistance in human health care. FEMS Microbiol Lett 363

Van der Meer Y (2017) Nutrition of pigs kept under low and high sanitary conditions: effects on animo acid and energy metabolism and damaging behaviour. p. 182. WUR Wageningen

Veldman KT, Wit B, Franz E, Wullings B, Heederik D & Mevius DJ (2020) Monitoring of Antimicrobial Resistance and antibiotic usage in animals in The Netherlands in 2019. pp. 80. Bioveterinary Research (WBVR) Lelystad

Veldman KT, Wit B, Franz E, Heederik DJJ (2024) Maran 2024 monitoring of antimicrobial resistance and antibiotic usage in animals in The Netherlands in 2023. Wageningen Bioveterinary Research, Wageningen, p 77

Visser K, Rommers J, Ipema B, Verkaik J, Gerritzen M & Van Reenen K (2015) Risicoanalyse dierenwelzijn zuivelketen. p. 78

Walsh F, Duffy B (2013) The culturable soil antibiotic resistome: a community of multi-drug resistant bacteria. PLoS One 8:e65567

Wilhelm B, Rajic A, Parker S, Waddell L, Sanchez J, Fazil A, Wilkins W, McEwen SA (2012) Assessment of the efficacy and quality of evidence for five on-farm interventions for Salmonella reduction in grow-finish swine: a systematic review and meta-analysis. Prev Vet Med 107:1–20

Zhou K, Zhou L, Lim Q, Zou R, Stephanopoulos G, Too HP (2011) Novel reference genes for quantifying transcriptional responses of Escherichia coli to protein overexpression by quantitative PCR. BMC Mol Biol 12:18

Chapter 7
Enforcement of the EU Regulations 2019/4 and 2019/6

Benno ter Kuile

Abstract This chapter is a selection of the articles from regulations EU 2019/4 and EU 2019/6 that are relevant for antibiotics policies with a short comment on law enforcement aspects. For a scientist it is nice to notice that the regulation matches the scientific insights of the time they were drafted and adopted. The enforcement may be straightforward or require a further filling in of open standards.

Keywords Law enforcement on AMR · Open standards · Veterinary medicine · AMR policy

Regulation 2019/4

Article 7 Cross-Contamination

1. Feed business operators manufacturing, storing, transporting or placing on the market medicated feed or intermediate products shall apply measures in accordance with Article 4 to avoid cross-contamination.

   Open standard; there are no clear demands on these measures.

2. The Commission is empowered to adopt delegated acts in accordance with Article 20 in order to supplement this Regulation by establishing specific maximum levels of cross-contamination for active substances in non-target feed, unless such levels are already established in accordance with Directive 2002/32/EC. Those delegated acts may also set out methods of analysis for active substances in feed.

   Maximum levels should be enforced. No room for interpretation.

B. ter Kuile (✉)
Department of Molecular Biology and Microbial Food Safety, Swammerdam Institute of Life Sciences, University of Amsterdam, Amsterdam, The Netherlands

Netherlands Food and Consumer Product Safety Authority, Utrecht, The Netherlands
e-mail: b.h.terkuile@uva.nl

B. ter Kuile (ed.), *Antimicrobial Resistance and Antibiotics Usage in Livestock*,
https://doi.org/10.1007/978-3-032-04598-0_7

Article 11 Advertising of Medicated Feed and Intermediate Products

1. The advertising of medicated feed and intermediate products shall be prohibited. That prohibition shall not apply to advertising made exclusively to veterinarians.

   Only advertisement aimed at farmers would be relevant and prohibited.

2. The advertising shall not include information in any form which could be misleading or lead to incorrect use of the medicated feed.

   Open standard: what is misleading?

3. Medicated feed shall not be distributed for promotional purposes except for small quantities of samples.
4. Medicated feed containing antimicrobial veterinary medicinal products shall not be distributed for promotional purposes as samples or in any other presentation.

   An exception on paragraph 3 for antibiotics.

Article 16 Prescription

5. By way of derogation from point (h) of Article 3(2) and paragraph 2 of this Article, a Member State may allow a veterinary prescription for medicated feed to be issued by a professional person qualified to do so in accordance with applicable national law on 27 January 2019.

   Such prescriptions shall exclude prescription of medicated feed containing antimicrobial veterinary medicinal products or any other veterinary medicinal products where a diagnosis by a veterinarian is necessary and shall be valid only in that Member State.

   Only a veterinarian can prescribe medicated feed with antibiotics. To be enforced as stated.

8. The veterinary prescription for medicated feed shall be valid from the date of its issuance for a maximum period of six months for non-food-producing animals other than fur animals and three weeks for food-producing animals and fur animals. In the case of medicated feed containing antimicrobial veterinary medicinal products, the prescription shall be valid from the date of its issuance for a maximum period of five days.

   Another exception of antibiotics: only 5 days validity of the prescription.

9. The veterinarian issuing the veterinary prescription for medicated feed shall verify that that medication is justified for the target animals on veterinary grounds. Furthermore that veterinarian shall ensure that the administration of the veteri-

nary medicinal product concerned is not incompatible with another treatment or use and that there is no contra-indication or interaction where several medicinal products are used. In particular, the veterinarian shall not prescribe medicated feed with more than one veterinary medicinal product containing antimicrobials.

This paragraph can be used to call a veterinarian who incorrectly prescribes antibiotics to order. The last sentence prohibits prescribing feed with two antibiotics at the same time, unless these together form a medicinal product that has been admitted.

Article 17 Use of Medicated Feed

3. Medicated feed containing antimicrobial veterinary medicinal products shall be used in accordance with Article 107 of Regulation (EU) 2019/6, except as regards paragraph 3 thereof, and shall not be used for prophylaxis.

This article forbids the use of medicated feed as prophylaxis. To be enforced as stated.

Annex IV Permitted Tolerances for the Compositional Labelling of Medicated Feed or Intermediate Products as Referred to in Article 9(3)

Where the composition of a medicated feed or an intermediate product is found to deviate from the amount of an antimicrobial active substance indicated on the label, a tolerance of 10% shall apply.

No room for interpretation. Enforce as stated.

Regulation 2019/6

Article 34 Classification of Veterinary Medicinal Products

1. The competent authority or the Commission, as applicable, granting a marketing authorisation as referred to in Article 5(1) shall classify the following veterinary medicinal products as subject to veterinary prescription:

(c) antimicrobial veterinary medicinal products;

Antibiotics may only be prescribed by veterinarians; Enforce as stated.

Article 35 Summary of the Product Characteristics

1. The summary of the product characteristics referred to in point (a) of Article 33(1) shall contain, in the order indicated below, the following information:

(xii) special conditions for use, including restrictions on the use of antimicrobial and antiparasitic veterinary medicinal products in order to limit the risk of development of resistance;

Check if this information is indeed provided

Article 37 Decisions Refusing Marketing Authorisations

3. A marketing authorisation for an antimicrobial veterinary medicinal product shall be refused if the antimicrobial is reserved for treatment of certain infections in humans as provided for in paragraph 5.
4. The Commission shall adopt delegated acts in accordance with Article 147 in order to supplement this Regulation by establishing the criteria for the designation of the antimicrobials which are to be reserved for treatment of certain infections in humans in order to preserve the efficacy of those antimicrobials.
5. The Commission shall, by means of implementing acts, designate antimicrobials or groups of antimicrobials reserved for treatment of certain infections in humans. Those implementing acts shall be adopted in accordance with the examination procedure referred to in Article 145(2).

   These paragraphs are about the critically important antibiotics for use in human health care. Application of these compounds for treating infections in livestock is prohibited. At the moment of writing this list, that is updated regularly, contains the (fluoro)quinolones, third generation and higher cephalosporins, macrolides, ketolides, glycopeptides and polymyxins, such as colistin. Strict enforcement of this rule is essential to prevent unnecessary development of these essential antibiotics.

Article 57 Collection of Data on Antimicrobial Medicinal Products Used in Animals

1. Member States shall collect relevant and comparable data on the volume of sales and on the use of antimicrobial medicinal products used in animals, to enable in particular the direct or indirect evaluation of the use of such products in food-producing animals at farm level, in accordance with this Article and within the time limits set out in paragraph 5.

2. Member States shall send collated data on the volume of sales and the use per animal species and per types of antimicrobial medicinal products used in animals to the Agency in accordance with paragraph 5 and within the time limits referred to therein. The Agency shall cooperate with Member States and with other Union agencies to analyse those data and shall publish an annual report. The Agency shall take into account those data when adopting any relevant guidelines and recommendations.

This article deals with the obligation of the member states to collect data on sales and usage of antimicrobials.

Article 105 Veterinary Prescriptions

1. A veterinary prescription for an antimicrobial medicinal product for metaphylaxis shall only be issued after a diagnosis of the infectious disease by a veterinarian.

   Enforcement is complicated by the fact that a single infected animal within a group is in principle enough to justify prescribing antibiotics.

2. The veterinarian shall be able to provide justification for a veterinary prescription of antimicrobial medicinal products, in particular for metaphylaxis and for prophylaxis.

   Enforcement a3ccording to the statement.

4. By way of derogation from point (33) of Article 4 and paragraph 3 of this Article, a Member State may allow a veterinary prescription to be issued by a professional, other than a veterinarian, who is qualified to do so in accordance with applicable national law at the time of entry into force of this Regulation. Such prescriptions shall be valid only in that Member State and shall exclude prescriptions of antimicrobial medicinal products and any other veterinary medicinal products where a diagnosis by a veterinarian is necessary.

   Again, only the veterinarian can prescribe antibiotics.

6. The quantity of the medicinal products prescribed shall be limited to the amount required for the treatment or therapy concerned. As regards antimicrobial medicinal products for metaphylaxis or prophylaxis, they shall be prescribed only for a limited duration to cover the period of risk.

   The problem is that suppliers of antimicrobials often offer only a limited number of sizes, e.g. 1 or 5 kilo. In that case the farmer is left with unneeded antibiotics. Proper disposal is complex.

10. A veterinary prescription for antimicrobial medicinal products shall be valid for 5 days from the date of its issue.

    Enforcement according to the statement.

11. In addition to the requirements set out in this Article, Member States may lay down rules on record-keeping for veterinarians when issuing veterinary prescriptions.

This authority to force veterinarians to keep proper records is an important tool for monitoring antibiotic usage.

Article 107 Use of Antimicrobial Medicinal Products

1. Antimicrobial medicinal products shall not be applied routinely nor used to compensate for poor hygiene, inadequate animal husbandry or lack of care or to compensate for poor farm management.

   This is an important paragraph for law enforcement agencies, as it empowers them to demand improvements when the abovementioned shortcomings are noticed and cause an increased usage of antimicrobials. The standards are open, so the competent authorities must formulate clear policies on these issues in advance.

2. Antimicrobial medicinal products shall not be used in animals for the purpose of promoting growth nor to increase yield.

   Strict enforcement of the ban on the use of antimicrobials as growth promoters is essential for limiting development and spreading of antimicrobial resistance. Application of antibiotics in low doses is suspicious.

3. Antimicrobial medicinal products shall not be used for prophylaxis other than in exceptional cases, for the administration to an individual animal or a restricted number of animals when the risk of an infection or of an infectious disease is very high and the consequences are likely to be severe.

   Prophylaxis is usually only allowed in special cases, such as before an operation.

In such cases, the use of antibiotic medicinal products for prophylaxis shall be limited to the administration to an individual animal only, under the conditions laid down in the first subparagraph.

   Even when needed for a specific reason, group prophylaxis treatment is forbidden

4. Antimicrobial medicinal products shall be used for metaphylaxis only when the risk of spread of an infection or of an infectious disease in the group of animals is high and where no other appropriate alternatives are available. Member States may provide guidance regarding such other appropriate alternatives and shall actively support the development and application of guidelines which promote the understanding of risk factors associated with metaphylaxis and include criteria for its initiation.

Metaphylaxis is only allowed as risk reducing measure and even then guidelines are to be observed. These guidelines can be drafted by, or under supervision of, the member states.

5. Medicinal products which contain the designated antimicrobials referred to in Article 37(5) shall not be used in accordance with Articles 112, 113 and 114.

   This paragraph rules out the veterinary use of antimicrobials critically important for human health care.

6. The Commission may, by means of implementing acts, and taking into consideration scientific advice of the Agency, establish a list of antimicrobials which:

   (a) shall not be used in accordance with Articles 112, 113 and 114; or
   (b) shall only be used in accordance with Articles 112, 113 and 114 subject to certain conditions.

   When adopting those implementing acts, the Commission shall take account of the following criteria:

   (a) risks to animal or public health if the antimicrobial is used in accordance with Articles 112, 113 and 114;
   (b) risk for animal or public health in case of development of antimicrobial resistance;
   (c) availability of other treatments for animals;
   (d) availability of other antimicrobial treatments for humans;
   (e) impact on aquaculture and farming if the animal affected by the condition receives no treatment.

   Those implementing acts shall be adopted in accordance with the examination procedure referred to in Article 145(2).

   This paragraph grants the Commission the authority to allow veterinary use of certain antimicrobials that normally would be exempted from livestock applications.

7. A Member State may further restrict or prohibit the use of certain antimicrobials in animals on its territory if the administration of such antimicrobials to animals is contrary to the implementation of a national policy on prudent use of antimicrobials.
8. Measures adopted by the Member States on the basis of paragraph 7 shall be proportionate and justified.
9. The Member State shall inform the Commission of any measure it has adopted on the basis of paragraph 7.

Paragraphs 7, 8 and 9 create the possibility for member states to prohibit use of certain antibiotics that they judge essential for human use due to particular considerations valid for their situation. If they choose to do so, they must report this to the EU Commission with a ground for this decision.

Article 118 Animals or Products of Animal Origin Imported into the Union

1. Article 107(2) shall apply, mutatis mutandis, to operators in third countries and those operators shall not use the designated antimicrobials referred to in Article 37(5), insofar as relevant in respect of animals or products of animal origin exported from such third countries to the Union.
2. The Commission shall adopt delegated acts in accordance with Article 147 in order to supplement this Article by providing the necessary detailed rules on the application of paragraph 1 of this Article.

The first paragraph prohibits import of animals raised with growth promoters and of foodstuffs of animal origin when the animals have been treated with antibiotics that are reserved for human health care. The second paragraph authorizes the Commission to fill in the details. The article aims at preventing the introduction of unwanted forms of resistance via animals or foodstuffs of animal origin. For law enforcement the proof may be complicated as resistance against an antibiotics does not prove it has been applied. Possibly patterns of resistance can be a ground for suspicion.

Article 152 Existing Veterinary Medicinal Products, Marketing Authorisations and Registrations

1. Marketing authorisations of veterinary medicinal products and registrations of homeopathic veterinary medicinal products granted in accordance with Directive 2001/82/EC or Regulation (EC) No 726/2004 before 28 January 2022 shall be deemed to have been issued in accordance with this Regulation, and are, as such, subject to the relevant provisions of this Regulation.

   The first subparagraph of this paragraph shall not apply to marketing authorisations for antimicrobial veterinary medicinal products containing antimicrobials which have been reserved for treatment in humans in accordance with implementing acts referred to in Article 37(5).

Antibiotics reserved for human use may not be marketed and used based on an old license granted before 28 January 2022, while all other veterinary medicines may.